CURE THE CAUSES
COOK BOOK

CURE THE CAUSES
COOK BOOK

Dr. Christina Rahm

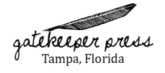

gatekeeper press
Tampa, Florida

Cure the Causes Cookbook

Published by Gatekeeper Press
7853 Gunn Hwy, Suite 209
Tampa, FL 33626
www.GatekeeperPress.com

The cover design, interior formatting, typesetting, and editorial work for this book are entirely the product of the author. Gatekeeper Press did not participate in and is not responsible for any aspect of these elements.

Library of Congress Control Number: 2022950470

ISBN (hardcover): 9781662934117
ISBN (paperback): 9781662934124
eISBN: 9781662934131

Contents

Acknowledgments

I want to thank my parents and grandparents for helping me learn how to cook. I used to think I might grow up to be a famous chef, but that didn't happen. However, I did grow up working on various formulations, inventions, and patents that helped people from a health and wellness perspective.

I believe the nutritional supplements I have worked on have helped so many people. But I also believe the food I cook helps people too! I know my grandmother's, my grandfather's, and my mother's food helped me feel good, even though I wasn't sick. The food they made also brought me joy as it went from my mouth to my stomach. I still miss eating their food. When I taste food like the food my family made me growing up, my mind immediately goes back to fond memories of love and joy. Even the smell of food can do this to me! So, a special thanks to all the amazing family members and friends that have fed me!!

Our bodies are cities inside. The brain, stomach, and heart are all connected, just like different areas of a city are connected. Our cells communicate inside. Our cells need to be protected and supported, just like the people in a city. We are in charge of the inside of our bodies, and we have to give our bodies the nutrients and food it needs.

Thank you to Clay, Ted, Patrick, Tyger, Jayla, Alice, Stephanie, Tiffany, Nicole, Alice, Leslie, Kline, Steve, Nicholas, Preston, Andy, Matt, Dr. Tina, Dr. Dori, Dr. K and Z, the ISNS Drs. and advisors, the people at the ROOT brands, the individuals behind Dr. Christina Rahm, LLC., and the founders of Cure the Causes for being behind me, helping with edits, and for your support. And as always, special thanks to my children, Duquesne, Merritt Ella, Crider "Roo," and Presto! Without you, my life would not be complete.

Medical Disclaimer

The information provided is for educational purposes only and is not intended as medical advice or a substitute for the medical advice of a physician or other qualified health care professionals.

This information is not to be used for self-diagnosis. Always consult your doctor for medical advice or information about diagnosis and treatment.

Statements have not been evaluated by the Food and Drug Administration (FDA).

Introduction

If you are health conscious and want to learn to treat your body well, this book is for you. Taking this a step further, this book is for people that strive for the ultimate mission of greatness for the inside and outside of their bodies and lives. As a scientist, I do not ever claim to cure diseases and illnesses, instead, I educate on natural ways to assist your bodies in dealing with the various environmental attacks that occur in life.

This book shows how you can support your body naturally by getting to the root of the issues that cause the various wars and illnesses that occur inside of our bodies. Environmental factors like viruses, bacteria, parasites, fungus, inflammation, stress, and anxiety can cause major problems to our bodies and lives. BUT there are answers and solutions, and I will share some of these in the book.

This book was written with the goal of helping teach people how to naturally support their bodies by using various types of plants, vegetables, fruits, proteins, and foods that support the body when it is dealing with various types of physical and mental health issues—ranging from cancer and arthritis to depression, autism, and other health problems. Moreover, the book also shares plenty of recipes to help you learn how you can assist your body in dealing with different types of diseases by making healthier eating choices. Every chapter discusses a specific list of ailments and showcases natural remedies that can assist people and their bodies by eradicating things outside of the body and optimizing the nutrients inside of the body. By doing what is right for the body, we can assist the body with reducing inflammation and can help people successfully manage health and disease-related medical complications. For example, if there is a chapter about fungal growth, not only will you find useful information about what type of disease it is, its symptoms and diagnosis, but also about the type of foods you can eat to assist the body at getting to the cause of this overgrowth and help the body self-heal or prevent further complications of ailments. At the end of every chapter, some recipes are shared to help you cook organic foods that aid your body in fighting infections, viruses, fungus, and various types of bacteria.

Remember, your body is your home, where you must live until it ceases to function. This book will teach you some valuable lessons related to dealing with your body in a friendly way. In other words, provide it with the best nutrients so that it gains the strength and resistance to fight off illnesses and other serious medical complications.

When your body is strong and resilient, it can even help you fight cancer. Since cancer is a life-threatening illness, its treatment is also tough for the body to resist. Both the disease and the treatment need your body to be strong, so you can fight back. When you have a compromised immune system, it will get very difficult for your body to fight back. When your immune system is strong, it is easier for you to fight back. If you already have healthy eating habits and you are keen on taking good care of your body, you can help it survive any battle.

Healthy living is all about enjoying your life, no matter how long you live. If you go on to live for a hundred years but are always sick and unhealthy, it is not as enjoyable, due to poor quality of life. However, if you live for fifty years or so with a healthier and stronger body, capable of resisting the worst ailments, you have more opportunities to enjoy your life and love your life.

I want people to enjoy their lives. I want people to be happy and healthy. Each person matters in this world. I hope this book helps you and the others around you to have a healthier and happier life!

Prologue

I was sick a lot as a child. I had a lot of allergies and illnesses. Then, when I was about 19, I contracted Lyme disease and I lost many parts of my memory. This was hard for me because memories and the ability to learn are important parts of living. I had to grow up quick. I realized that no one ever promised us life would be easy. Our bodies are not perfect. Life is not perfect. We are surrounded by illnesses, stress, diseases, viruses, parasites, bacteria, fungus, heavy metals, and pollution. Genetics become epigenetics, and many of us get very sick during this transition.

I realize now that I was given a type of gift to get sick after I had my oldest son. It taught me to grow up and live each day to its fullest. It also taught me how important it was to take care of myself. Having multiple doctorate degrees in various forms of psychological, scientific, and nutritional areas, these have not been what has motivated me to learn and teach about nutrition and food. I did love this part of my education, but this desire I have to touch and teach people through food and diet is predominantly because of what I have personally been through in my life.

I hope this helps your life and soul survive. Great food and nutritional food is undervalued. Its importance is much higher than most of us realize. Here's a toast to your life and the food you eat. I hope it is better and greater after reading this book!

Dr. Christina Rahm

CHAPTER 1

Nutritional Recipes to Support Autoimmune Disorders

There are more than 80 novel autoimmune diseases. However, what they share, for all intents and purposes, is a failing of the body's immunity. Our bodies need to support the good cells and get rid of the bad cells, but unfortunately this does not happen correctly when your body has an autoimmune impairment. A few autoimmune disorders target only one organ, and others focus on the entire body. While specialists don't know precisely everything that causes each autoimmune disease, they do know that certain individuals have a higher rate of expectancy, due to genetics and environmental factors. Women are twice as likely as men to experience the ill effects of autoimmune diseases, particularly during childbearing years (ages 15 to 44). Also, certain autoimmune diseases generally run-in families or influence specific cultural groups more. The 12 most common autoimmune diseases (recorded here from most noteworthy pervasiveness) are:

- Autoimmune thyroiditis (Hashimoto's thyroiditis and different sorts): influences the thyroid, making it over- or under-produce hormones that influence digestion

- Psoriasis: influences skin cells, making them increase too rapidly

- Rheumatoid joint inflammation influences the joints

- Type 1 diabetes: influences insulin-delivering cells in the pancreas

- Multiple sclerosis: influences the defensive covering around nerve cells and the focal sensory system

- Ulcerative colitis: an inflammatory gut sickness influencing the internal organ and rectum

- Celiac illness: influences the gastrointestinal parcel when gluten is ingested

- Systemic lupus erythematosus influences numerous organs, including joints, kidneys, cerebrum, heart, and skin

- Myasthenia gravis: influences nerve motivations that help the mind control muscles

- Systemic sclerosis: influences the skin and connective tissue

- Sjogren's disorder: influences glands that oil up the eyes and mouth

- Crohn's disease: an inflammatory entrail infection influencing any piece of the gastrointestinal tract

Symptoms of autoimmune diseases are comparative and profoundly individualized. A similar condition can appear in certain pathological ways among various individuals and present completely different in other individuals. Early symptoms of autoimmune circumstances can include exhaustion and disarray, aches and deadness in areas of the body, balding, skin rashes, inflammation, and severe fever.

For most people, it is important to consult an expert. Experts can help us diagnose and treat autoimmune diseases. Often, you will need a team to help you. I believe that one opinion is not enough, and various approaches should be explored. Treatments, as a rule, include medications that focus on the eruption and symptoms of the autoimmune disorders. Nutrition is also an aspect that needs to be reviewed and you should have plans that are put together. It is important to distinguish any food that could make autoimmune disorder or symptoms worse. It is also imperative to get rid of any trigger food sources, medications, or environmental factors that make health and living worse. For example, Type 1 diabetes is a case where hyper and hypoglycemia (too high glucose and too low glucose) can be controlled with a mix of glucose monitoring and insulin. Nonetheless, another way of assisting the body during these treatments is by making positive changes, like nutritious eating, diet, and supplements. Western and Eastern medicine can also be incorporated, as the main goal is to help control Type 1 diabetes and bring the body to healing and greatness.

What to Eat to Help Control Autoimmune Sickness

Nutritious eating intended to control or lessen eruptions related to various autoimmune diseases ought to be individualized. Working with a medical services supplier or enrolled dietitian with some expertise in your autoimmune condition can help you decide the best methodology for you. For instance, individuals with ulcerative colitis and Crohn's sickness might experience issues eating crude vegetables and organic products. They would have to utilize elective ways to incorporate such food varieties into their eating regimen (like cooking, puréeing, and squashing for simpler processing). A few other healthful treatments for autoimmune diseases include:

Gluten-Free diet: A strict gluten-free diet is fundamental for individuals with celiac illness. In this autoimmune condition, ingesting even limited quantities of gluten can trigger an insusceptible reaction that attacks the covering of the digestive tract. Gluten appears in items containing wheat or wheat subsidiaries, grain, rye, or triticale. Individuals with other autoimmune circumstances, like psoriasis or Hashimoto's thyroiditis, may encounter fewer outbursts when on a gluten-free diet. However, a few circumstances might worsen, contingent upon the general refreshing effect of the gluten-free diet (it's important to stress entire and new gluten-free food sources versus bundled and handled gluten-free food sources, for instance).

Anti-Inflammatory diet: During a resistant reaction, there is an expansion in the creation of free radicals, which can bring about an awkwardness of support of oxidants to antioxidants, known as oxidative pressure. Therefore, an eating approach loaded with anti-inflammatory and antioxidant food varieties while killing realized inflammatory food varieties, could be advantageous at turning around the oxidative pressure that accompanies many sorts of autoimmune circumstances. This style is like a Mediterranean diet that inclines intensely on new produce, entire grains, and solid fats from fish, olives, and nuts. Study "eating to beat inflammation."

Plant-Based diet: A diet that stresses all (veggie lover) or generally (vegan) plant-based food sources has been associated with higher antioxidant consumption, which can help individuals with autoimmune circumstances. Plant-based diets revolve around food sources that consist mostly of plant-based foods such as—beans, vegetables, organic products, nuts, seeds, grains, and plant-determined oils.

Autoimmune protocol (AIP): This temporary eating strategy is like the paleo diet and includes a few periods of end and renewed introduction of specific food varieties, to recognize triggers. Wiped-out food sources frequently incorporate espresso, oils, liquor, grains, dairy, eggs, vegetables, nuts, seeds, nightshade vegetables, refined sugars, and tobacco, and that's only the tip of the iceberg. During this stage (which commonly endures 1 to 90 days), the accentuation is on new products, insignificantly handled meat and fish, aged food varieties, and bone stock. After the end stage, food varieties are deliberately and gradually introduced, generally each, in turn, observing any responses.

Food Sources to Lessen When You Have Autoimmune Infection:

Straightforward sugars: Foods that contain added sugars or high fructose corn syrup, as well as food varieties that are profoundly handled and high in starch (white bread and pasta, cereals, cakes, and prepared merchandise), have been associated with expanded aggravation. These food sources are usually low in fiber and other gainful supplements.

Certain oils: Vegetable oils (vegetable mixes, soybean oil, and corn oil) and seed oils (cottonseed, sunflower seed, and sesame oil) in addition to nut oil, palm oil, and rice grain oil have a high proportion of omega-6 unsaturated fats to omega-3 unsaturated fats, which has been connected to persistent irritation. These oils are modest and synthetically separated, appearing in many exceptionally handled food sources.

Trans fats: Everyone ought to lessen or dispose of trans fats for, generally speaking, well-being. This is particularly valid for individuals with autoimmune infection, since trans unsaturated fats are undoubtedly connected with irritation. The FDA has restricted fake trans fats; however, food varieties that contain under 0.5 grams of trans fat per serving can list 0 grams of trans fat on the "Nutrition Facts" label. While this sum is small, it can add up rapidly. Trans fats exist mostly in bundled prepared merchandise, a few margarine and vegetable shortenings, some microwave popcorns, broiled cheap food, non-dairy flavors, refrigerated batters, and bread rolls. Assuming an item contains "to some extent hydrogenated oil" is a decent sign it has trans fats.

Processed meat: Advanced glycation results (AGEs) in processed meats, like wieners franks, and store meats are known to cause irritation and might be particularly triggering for ulcerative colitis and Crohn's sickness.

Dairy: People with autoimmune illnesses respond adversely to lactose, a characteristic sugar in dairy, and have fewer symptoms when dairy is restricted. Foods most advanced in lactose include cow's milk, cream, frozen yogurt, and delicate cheeses like spreadable cheddar, Brie, Camembert, cottage cheese, and mozzarella cheese.

Unreasonable alcohol: Research shows that over-the-top liquor utilization is frequently connected with a "leaky tummy," which can move irritation from the colon into different body parts. Keep away from liquor totally or restrict it to two beverages or less each day for men and one beverage or less each day for women, which is identical to 12 ounces of beer, 5 ounces of wine, or 1.5 ounces of 80-proof spirits.

Supplements That Can Help with Autoimmune Disease:

Extra support from specific supplements could help decrease or reduce a resistant reaction in individuals with autoimmune illnesses. Continuously consult your doctor before beginning another enhancement.

Vitamin D: This nutrient helps keep the immune system working by reducing the creation of proinflammatory cytokines. Lack of vitamin D has been associated with a few autoimmune diseases, including multiple sclerosis and Type 1 diabetes. A few investigations show that ingesting 400 IUs or more each day can diminish the risk of a few autoimmune circumstances by 40%.

Prebiotics, probiotics, and symbiotics: A sound stomach and good microbiome can help neutralize the seriousness of a few autoimmune symptoms and forestall worsening "cracked stomach."

Omega 3s: The anti-inflammatory properties of EPA and DHA—two powerful omega-3 unsaturated fats—help oversee autoimmune diseases and are often suggested in treatments for rheumatoid joint pain, Crohn's illness, lupus erythematosus, and multiple sclerosis.

Anti-inflammatory supplements: Studies highlight intensifies in specific homegrown and green growth supplements as strong suppressors of favorable to inflammatory compounds, particularly curcumin, Boswellia, resveratrol, black cumin oil, ginger, and spirulina.

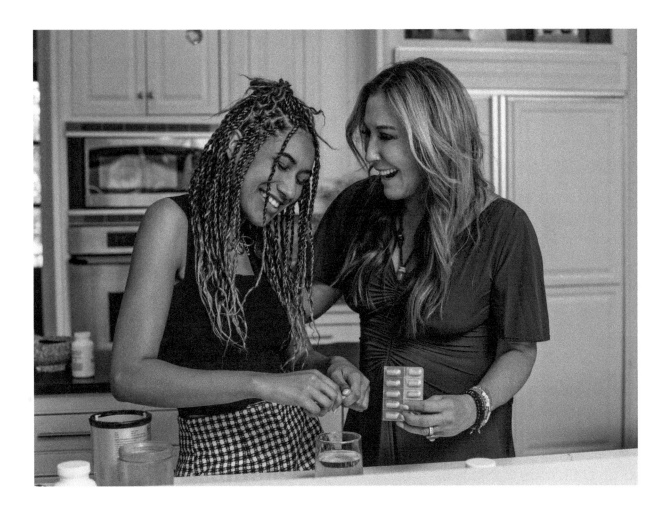

Have Autoimmune Illness? Do This First:

If you suspect you have an autoimmune disease but don't have a decision yet, begin there. Request a meeting with a medical care provider who spends significant time in autoimmune cases and is ready to access and diagnose through various meetings and examinations. Be prepared to talk about your symptoms and what you think could be some of the triggers. If you think you have an autoimmune disorder but it has not been diagnosed, begin by surrounding yourself with positive energy, getting plenty of sleep, drinking lots of water, limiting alcohol, and processed food sources, and using natural supplements that help you eradicate the toxins out of the body, while supporting the body in its fight against inflammation and illness.

What Else to Be Aware of with Autoimmune Disease?

Besides food, there are a few factors that can exacerbate autoimmune circumstances. Think about the suggested dietary methodologies presented above and review additional suggestions below:

Prescriptions: Suppliers might endorse NSAIDs or other supportive medications, since autoimmune circumstances frequently accompany intense or ongoing agony. NSAIDs should be avoided in the disposal period of an AIP diet, so examine this with your doctor, assuming you might want to attempt that methodology. Likewise, antibiotics can help treat a few autoimmune diseases, like Crohn's, but can adversely affect stomach microbiota. If an antibiotic is endorsed, get some information about following it with a probiotic or symbiotic (a probiotic + prebiotic formula).

Get some rest: Sleep issues, including exhaustion, a sleeping disorder, and daytime lethargy, are many times an admonition indication of autoimmune illness. Also, not getting sufficient rest can be further unsafe to the insusceptible framework. Laying out a normal rest plan (at the end of the week too) and loosening up a custom one hour before sleep time can help, as can seeing a rest subject matter expert.

Keep a diary: Keeping a diary to follow day-to-day food consumption, medicine, rest, mindset, stress, development, and more can be one of your most helpful tools in distinguishing any examples or triggers associated with the eruptions of your autoimmune sickness.

Do low-impact workouts: If you've encountered a fit, for example, the joint irritation and fatigue related to rheumatoid joint pain, you realize that it tends to be hard to work out. Yet, getting into a standard and every day development example can work on personal satisfaction with any autoimmune infection. Begin with low-impact exercises that are more straightforward on joints—like walking, yoga, or swimming—and add high-impact or cardio practices a couple of times each week.

Reduce environmental toxin exposure and smoking: Reductions in smoking tobacco or long-haul exposure to different toxins, like air and water contaminations, fine silica, bright radiation, or different solvents has been related to the improvement of autoimmune diseases, like multiple sclerosis and rheumatoid joint pain.

Autoimmune diseases, for example, rheumatoid joint swelling, lupus, and thyroid disorders are difficult, problematic, and frequently damaging. At their core, they practically share one thing: a crazy safe reaction connected with systemic irritation. The right diet can help ease torment and heal autoimmune diseases. As a rule, avoid caffeine, liquor, sugar, grains, dairy, and red meat, and spotlight natural products, vegetables, solid fats, and fish.

Which Food Sources Are Awesome for Helping and Mending Autoimmune Diseases?

Attempt these six food varieties to make living with autoimmune circumstances simpler:

Halibut

One 3-ounce serving of halibut has more than an entire day's worth of vitamin D, which is connected with the diminished risk of rheumatoid joint pain, multiple sclerosis, lupus, and other autoimmune diseases. Incorporating halibut into your meals can help you get your fill of vitamin D and possibly bring down your risk. Other great wellsprings of vitamin D include salmon, mackerel, sardines, whitefish, and fish. Choose egg yolks or mushrooms filled in daylight or UV light for vegan sources.

Attempt this: Marinate halibut steaks in olive oil and garlic, then barbecue until done and embellish with lemons and parsley; or layer halibut steaks with rosemary and shallots, envelop in parchment or foil and prepare until done; or poach halibut in white wine, cut into strips and serve on a plate of mixed greens of arugula, daintily cut fennel, orange portions, and dark olives.

Turmeric

This dazzling orange powder contains curcumin, a strong recuperating compound that has been displayed to mitigate multiple sclerosis, rheumatoid joint pain, psoriasis, and inflammatory entrail illness by directing inflammatory substances in the body. Turmeric is particularly gainful for battling aggravation, and examination shows that it might help mitigate some autoimmune or irritation-related symptoms.

In any case, curcumin is difficult for the body to absorb. To expand its accessibility, join it with black pepper and try heating it, the two practices combined make it simpler for the body to utilize.

Blend curry into a paste, then purée for a simple, smooth soup; or stew coconut or almond milk with turmeric and black pepper and improve with wild honey for dairy-free, golden milk; or toss cauliflower florets in turmeric, black pepper, salt, garlic, and olive oil, then broil until lightly brown and tender when poked with a fork.

Sauerkraut

Generally, aged sauerkraut is stacked with probiotics, which help balance the stomach microbiome and further develop the digestive tract's boundary work. These are two basic capacities in safeguarding against autoimmune circumstances. Concentrates show that individuals with rheumatoid joint pain who take probiotics feel a critical decrease in firmness, enlargement, torment, and irritation.

Other great dairy-free probiotic sources incorporate kimchi, matured vegetables, salted ginger, coconut yogurt with added probiotics, and water kefir.

Attempt this: Purée sauerkraut with mustard, horseradish, and wild honey for a lively sandwich spread; or barbecue chicken or turkey hot dog, cut from corner to corner, and serve on a bed of sauerkraut; or blend sauerkraut with ground carrots, daikon radish, and spinach for a simple side.

Green tea

Green tea can work wonders for irritation and is intense nourishment for autoimmune diseases. This tea is high in a compound called epigallocatechin-3-gallate (EGCG), which has been displayed to develop symptoms further and lessen the pathology in a few creature models of autoimmune diseases. The dysregulation of T cell work is a basic factor in improving autoimmune inflammatory diseases. Green tea certainly affects T cell work, particularly their separation, in a way that can favorably affect autoimmunity.

Attempt this: Brew green tea with mint, slices of ginger, and natural honey; or blend fermented green tea, bananas, and coconut milk, then freeze in a container.

Wild Alaskan salmon

Salmon is wealthy in omega-3 unsaturated fats, which decrease aggravation, regulate safe action, and safeguard against a few inflammatory and autoimmune diseases, including rheumatoid joint pain, Crohn's illness, ulcerative colitis, psoriasis, and multiple sclerosis. In any case, wild salmon isn't the main fish that is great for autoimmune mending. Fish, sardines, mackerel, and other greasy fish are likewise great wellsprings of omega-3 fats.

Attempt this: Simmer kelp noodles in stock with ginger and garlic, then top with bok choy, scallions, and fragmented cooked salmon. Or, in a food processor, combine salmon, leeks, zucchini, garlic, and onions, then pulse blend and form into patties and sauté in olive oil; or toss canned salmon with solid avocado halves, chopped kale, sliced carrots, and a simple salad dressing.

Broccoli

Like other sulfur-rich food varieties (cauliflower, radishes, cabbage, onions, kale), broccoli is wealthy in a strong antioxidant called glutathione, which might help reduce autoimmune diseases. It's key in subduing persistent irritation and safeguarding against oxidative pressure. Concentrates show glutathione status can be lessened by as much as half in individuals with autoimmune disorders.

Attempt this: Toss entire broccoli spears in olive oil, garlic, and red pepper flakes and grill until delicate; or cook broccoli, cauliflower, and leeks in stock, then purée until smooth for a rich, dairy-free soup. Or mash or shred broccoli stems, red cabbage, celery, green apples, and onions, add goldenraisins, and dress with mayonnaise, natural honey, and apple cider vinegar for a simple slaw.

Bone Broth Recipe (stovetop or Instant Pot)

Serving Size - 6 servings

INGREDIENTS

- 2 lbs. bones from a healthy source
- 2 chicken feet (optional)
- 1 gallon of water
- 2 tablespoons apple cider vinegar
- 1 onion
- 2 carrots
- 2 stalks of celery
- 1 tablespoon salt (optional)
- 1 teaspoon peppercorns (optional)
- herbs and spices to taste (optional)
- 2 cloves garlic (optional)
- 1 bunch parsley (optional)
- 1 teaspoon "Root Restore"

INSTRUCTIONS

1. If you are using raw bones, especially beef bones, it improves flavor to roast them in the oven first. I place them in a roasting pan and roast for 30 minutes at 350°F.
2. After roasting, place the bones in a large stock pot or the Instant Pot.
3. Pour cool filtered water and the vinegar over the bones. Let sit for 20 to 30 minutes in the cool water. The acid in the vinegar helps make the nutrients in the bones more available.
4. Rough chop the onion, carrots, and celery and add to the pot.
5. Add any salt, pepper, spices, or herbs, if using.
6. On the stovetop, bring the broth to a boil over medium to high heat. Once it has reached a vigorous boil, reduce to a simmer and simmer for about 5-7 minutes until done.
7. During the first few hours of simmering, you'll need to remove the impurities that float to the surface. A frothy/foamy layer will form, and it can be easily scooped off with a big spoon. Throw this part away. I typically check it every 20 minutes for the first 2 hours to remove this. Grass-fed and healthy animals will produce much less of this than conventional animals.
8. Simmer for 8 hours for fish broth, 24 hours for chicken, and 48 hours for beef.

9. During the last 30 minutes, add the garlic and parsley, if using.

10. Remove from heat and let cool slightly. Strain, using a fine mesh strainer, to remove all the bits of bone and vegetable. When cool enough, store in a gallon-size glass jar in the fridge for up to 5 days, or freeze for later use.

INSTANT POT

1. Add the garlic and parsley to the pot, if using. Place the lid on the pot, and set valve to seal.

2. Cook at high pressure for 2 hours, followed by either a quick release or natural pressure release. Either is fine.

3. Let cool slightly, strain, and store in a gallon-size glass jar in the fridge for up to 5 days, or freeze for later use.

Homemade Sauerkraut Recipe

INGREDIENTS

- 2 heads cabbage (about five lbs.)
- ¼ cup salt (see note below)
- 1 to 2 tablespoons caraway seeds (optional)
- ¼ of a capsule of "Root Zero-In"

INSTRUCTIONS

1. Get things clean—wash all equipment, work surfaces, and your hands with warm soapy water.

2. Slice the cabbage—remove the outer leaves and cores from cabbage. (Compost them, if you can!) Cut the cabbage into quarters, for easier slicing. Then, slice cabbage into very thin ribbons. If you have one, a food processor speeds up this process.

3. Add the salt—place the thinly sliced cabbage in a large bowl (make sure it is clean too!) Sprinkle the salt over it. Knead and squish the cabbage/salt with your hands for about ten minutes. At first, it won't seem like it is doing anything at all, but be patient. After a few minutes, the cabbage will start releasing liquid and by the end, there should be enough liquid brine to cover the cabbage in the crock or jar. Add the caraway seeds, if using, and "Zero-In" at this point.

4. Move it to the fermentation vessel—stuff the cabbage very tightly into the jars or fermentation crock. Pour any liquid from the bowl into the jar. If needed, add just enough water to make sure the water/brine covers the cabbage entirely. If the cabbage is fresh, no liquid may be needed, but don't worry if you have to add a little water.

5. Weigh and cover—add the fermentation weights and fermentation seal (or use the fermentation crock as directed). If you are using a basic mason jar, you can also do this by adding a smaller jar that fits just inside the lid of the mason jar, and cover both jars with a cloth and a rubber band.

6. Let it ferment—now you get to practice patience! Fermentation will begin within a day and take 2 to 5 weeks, depending on temperature and desired tartness. After 2 weeks, check for desired tartness. The sauerkraut is technically slightly fermented after only a few days, but the best flavor seems to be at the 2 to 3 week mark. Taste is the best measure here, so check it often and stop the ferment when you get the desired taste. Note: It is normal to see bubbles, white scum, or foam on top during the fermentation. You shouldn't see any actual mold, though. If you do, scrape it off the top, and make sure all the rest of the cabbage is fully submerged. All cabbage below the brine level should still be fine.

7. Cool it down–once fermented, it can be eaten right away, or it will store in the refrigerator for up to six months.

Enjoy! Sauerkraut is delicious on its own or added to salads, soups, or on top of meats.

NOTES

- The salt should be at a ratio of about 2%, by weight. If you have a digital scale, it is worth weighing the cabbage and the salt, if you want to get the perfect ratio for the brine. I find it easiest to weigh the cabbage (in grams) and then calculate 2% of the weight of the cabbage to use in salt. Any high-quality salt will work, but I find the best results when I use Mediterranean sea salt.

CHAPTER 2

Nutritional Diet to Support Anti-Cancer Regimen

Eating sufficient food to get the nutrients and calories you need isn't typically an issue when you're healthy. Most food approaches stress eating loads of vegetables, organic products, and whole grain items; restricting how much red meat you eat, particularly meats that are handled or high in fat; scaling back fat, sugar, liquor, and salt; and remaining at a healthy weight. Yet, while you're being treated for cancer, these things can be difficult, particularly if you make side impacts or simply don't feel good.

Great nourishment is particularly important, assuming you have cancer, because both the ailment and its treatments can impact your eating. They can likewise influence how your body endures specific foods and uses nutrients.

During cancer treatment, you could have to change your diet to assist with developing your fortitude and withstand the impacts of cancer and its treatment. This might mean eating things that aren't normally suggested when you are healthy. For example, you could require high-protein, fatty foods to keep your weight, or thick, cool foods like frozen yogurt or milkshakes, since sores in your mouth and throat make it hard to eat anything. The sort of cancer, your treatment, and any side influences you have should be considered, while attempting to sort out the most effective ways to get the sustenance your body needs.

Sustenance is important for all cancer patients, yet nourishment isn't just about devouring healthy foods and drinks: your body needs to absorb nutrients to profit from them.

The principal capability of the colon is to absorb electrolytes and liquid; however, colorectal cancers and their treatments might obstruct supplement absorption.

Results of chemotherapy treatment might include sickness, vomiting, loss of hunger, looseness of the bowels, or clogging—any of which present nutritional challenges during treatment. While numerous cancer patients are in danger of hunger and drying out, those with gastrointestinal cancers (which incorporates colorectal cancer) are significantly more liable to encounter some level of lack of healthy sustenance, which might influence a patient's capacity to finish treatment.

Seeking legitimate sustenance during treatment assists patients with keeping a healthy weight, bulk, and energy levels—all of which add to the capacity to endure cancer treatment and plan for survivorship.

Exact nutritional requirements during cancer treatment fluctuate according to each understanding's circumstance. Patients with previous circumstances, like heart disease or obesity, face unexpected challenges compared to those who start treatment in somewhat great health. Patients' necessities likewise differ according to where they are in the treatment cycle and the secondary effects they experience.

As a rule, cancer patients need to remain hydrated and eat healthy foods high in proteins, nutrients, cell reinforcements, and electrolytes to assist them with accomplishing satisfactory caloric requirements. Working with an expert dietitian who can assist you with addressing those necessities and monitoring your nutritional status throughout your treatment routine may decrease your chance of encountering nutritional lacks during treatment.

The nourishment needs of individuals with cancer fluctuate from one individual to another. Your cancer care group can assist you with recognizing your sustenance objectives and plan ways of assisting you with meeting them. Eating great while you're being treated for cancer could help you:

- Feel better
- Keep up your strength and energy
- Maintain your weight and your body's store of nutrients
- Better tolerate treatment-related side effects
- Lower your risk of infection

Heal and Recover Faster

Eating great means eating different foods to give your body nutrients to battle cancer. These nutrients include proteins, fats, carbohydrates, water, vitamins, and minerals.

Proteins: We want protein for development, to fix body tissue, and keep our safe frameworks healthy. When your body doesn't get sufficient protein, it could separate muscle for the fuel it needs. This takes more time to recover from sickness and can lower protection from infection. Individuals with cancer often need more protein than expected. After the medical procedure, chemotherapy, or radiation treatment, additional protein is typically expected to heal tissues and assist with battling the infection.

Great sources of protein incorporate fish, poultry, lean red meat, eggs, low-fat dairy items, nuts, nut margarine, dried beans, peas, lentils, and soy foods.

Fats: Fats assume an important part in nourishment. Fats and oils act as a rich wellspring of energy for the body. The body separates fats and uses them to store energy, protect body tissues, and transport a few kinds of vitamins through the blood.

You might have heard that a few fats are better for you than others. While considering the effects of fats on your heart and cholesterol level, pick monounsaturated (olive, canola, and nut oils) and polyunsaturated fats (these are tracked down predominantly in safflower, sunflower, corn, and flaxseed oils, and fish) more often than saturated fats or trans fats.

Saturated fats are mostly found in natural sources like meat and poultry, whole or reduced fat milk, cheddar, and margarine. Some vegetable oils like coconut, palm piece oil, and palm oil are saturated. Saturated fats can raise cholesterol and increase your risk for heart disease. Under 10% of your calories should come from saturated fat.

Most trans fats in our diets come from ground foods and heated products made with, to some degree, hydrogenated vegetable oil or vegetable shortening. These sources of trans fats have generally been eliminated from the food supply in the US. Trans fats are additionally found in a few animal products, similar to dairy items, in more modest amounts. Trans fats can raise bad cholesterol and lower great cholesterol. Keep away from trans fats, however much you can.

Carbohydrates: Carbohydrates are the body's key source of energy, and give the body the energy it needs for actual work and suitable organ ability. The best sources of carbohydrates are organic products, vegetables, and whole grains, which supply the required vitamins, minerals, fiber, and phytonutrients. (Phytonutrients are synthetics in plant-based foods that we don't need to live, yet that could advance health.)

Fiber is a piece of plant food that the body can't process. There are 2 sorts of fiber: Insoluble fiber assists with rapidly moving food waste out of the body, and soluble fiber dissolves with water in the stool to assist with keeping stool soft.

Different sources of carbohydrates include bread, potatoes, rice, spaghetti, pasta, oats, corn, peas, and beans. Desserts (sweets, candy, and beverages with sugar) can supply carbohydrates. However, these are not a good source of vitamins, minerals, or phytonutrients.

Water: Water and fluids are imperative to health. All body cells need water to work. On the off chance that you don't take in an adequate number of liquids, or assuming you lose liquids through retching or looseness of the bowels, you can get dried out (your body doesn't have as much liquid as it ought to). Assuming this occurs, the liquids and minerals that assist with keeping your body working can be perilously out of equilibrium. You get water from the foods you eat, yet an individual should likewise drink around four 8-ounce glasses of fluid every day to be certain that all the body cells get the liquid they need. You might require additional liquids assuming you're heaving, have loose bowels, or, regardless, of whether you're simply not eating a lot. Keep as a top priority that all fluids (soups, milk, even frozen yogurt, and gelatin) figure in with your liquid objectives.

Vitamins and minerals: Your body needs vitamins and minerals to help it appropriately utilize food's energy (calories). Most are found normally in foods, yet they are sold as pills and fluid supplements.

If you eat a balanced diet with adequate calories and protein, you will typically get a lot of vitamins and minerals. In any case, it very well may be difficult to eat a balanced diet while you're being treated for cancer, particularly if you have treatment side effects. If you truly do make side impacts, your doctor or dietitian might recommend an every day multivitamin and mineral supplement. Assuming your food admission has been restricted for a little while or months because of the effects of treatment, make certain to tell your doctor. You could be checked for nutrient or mineral insufficiencies.

If you're considering taking a supplement, make certain to examine this with your doctor first. Certain individuals with cancer take a lot of vitamins, minerals, and other dietary supplements to attempt to support their insusceptible framework or even obliterate cancer cells. Yet, some of these substances can be destructive, particularly when taken in huge dosages. Enormous portions of certain vitamins and minerals might make chemotherapy and radiation treatment less successful.

Suppose your doctor says it's OK to take a nutrient during treatment. It might be ideal to pick a supplement without 100 percent of the daily value (DV) of vitamins and minerals and one without iron (except if your doctor thinks you want iron).

Antioxidants: Antioxidants incorporate vitamins A, C, and E, selenium, zinc, and a few proteins that absorb and join to free radicals (harmful particles), keeping them from going after normal cells.

To take in more antioxidants, health specialists suggest eating different foods grown from the ground, which are great sources of antioxidants. Taking enormous dosages of cell-support supplements, nutrient-boosted foods, or fluids is typically not suggested while seeking chemo or radiation treatment. Converse with your doctor to figure out the best opportunity to take cell-reinforcement supplements.

Phytonutrients: Phytonutrients or phytochemicals are plants chemicals like carotenoids, lycopene, resveratrol, and phytosterols that are known to have health-safeguarding characteristics. They're found in plants, like products of the soil or things produced using plants, similar to tofu or tea. Phytochemicals are best taken in by eating the foods that contain them instead of taking supplements or pills.

Spices: Spices have been utilized to treat disease for many years, with blended results. Today spices are found in numerous items, similar to pills, fluid concentrates, teas, and salves. Many of these items are innocuous and protected, yet others can cause dangerous side effects. Some might try and slow down cancer treatments and recovery from a medical procedure. If you're keen on utilizing items containing spices, discuss it with your cancer doctor, medical caretaker, or drug specialist first.

Dietary Supplement Well-Being Considerations

Many individuals accept that a pill or supplement they find in stores is protected and works. The Food and Drug Administration (FDA) has decided to assist with guaranteeing that supplements contain what their labels promise. However, the supplement's security and effects on the body are not tended to by any FDA rules. The FDA doesn't make producers of these items print possible side effects on their labels. And the FDA can't pull a dietary supplement or homegrown item from the market, except if they have proof that the item is difficult.

It's likewise been shown that numerous homegrown items aren't what the name says. A few items don't contain any of the ingredients they're supposed to. Some additionally contain possibly unsafe medications, added substances, or pollutants that aren't recorded on the label. This implies there's no certain method for knowing whether a supplement is protected or what it will mean for you.

Tell your cancer care group about any over-the-counter items or supplements you're using or are pondering. Take the bottle(s) to your doctor to discuss the portion, and ensure that the ingredients don't disrupt your health or cancer treatments.

What you eat is truly important when you have cancer. Your body needs an adequate number of calories and nutrients to remain solid. Be that as it may, the disease can make it hard to get what you want, which can be different before, during, and after treatment. And now and again, you actually won't feel like eating.

You needn't bother with an amazing diet makeover. A couple of basic tips can make great-for-you foods simple and tempting.

Before treatment

Begin zeroing in on healthy foods, even before you start your treatment. You don't know what it will mean for you or what side effects you could have. That is the reason it's really smart to get great sustenance now. It can assist you with feeling better and giving your body areas of strength for stay.

It's likewise a great chance to make arrangements for the days when you won't feel like making anything to eat. Fill your cooler and storage room with healthy foods that need very little (or no) cooking. Simple choices include nuts, fruit purée, yogurt, pre-cut veggies, and microwaveable earthy-colored rice, or other entire grains. Make groups of a portion of your favorite courses and freeze them.

You may likewise need to arrange a few loved ones who can bring you dinners for the main days or long stretches of your treatment.

During Treatment

You might have days when you feel hungry and when food is the last thing you need. On great days, eat heaps of protein and healthy calories. That will keep your body solid and assist with fixing harm from your treatment.

High-protein foods include:

- Lean meat, chicken, and fish
- Eggs
- Beans, nuts, and seeds
- Cheddar cheese, milk, and yogurt

Try to eat no less than 2 1/2 cups of food grown from the ground daily. Incorporate dull greens, strong yellow veggies, and organic citrus products, like oranges and grapefruits. Colorful foods like these have numerous healthy nutrients. Simply make certain to wash them thoroughly.

Drink a lot of fluids daily. Water is an incredible decision. Attempt new-pressed juice, as well, giving you a few additional vitamins alongside the fluid your body needs to remain hydrated.

It's additionally important that you don't eat raw or half-cooked meat, fish, and poultry. Try not to eat foods or drink refreshments that are unpasteurized. Eat when you're hungry. Assuming that it is in the morning, make breakfast your greatest feast—drink meal substitutions later, on the off chance that your hunger blurs as the day continues. If feasts are a battle, eat five or six little meals rather than a few major ones during the day. Have little, healthy tidbits on hand as well. Yogurt, grain, cheddar cheese, saltines, and soup are great decisions. If you're having chemotherapy, a bite or little dinner just before a meeting could keep sickness away.

Control Side Effects

Many side effects of cancer treatments can make it hard to get enough to eat. Your diet might assist you with moving beyond probably the most widely recognized issues.

- *Nausea/vomiting:* Avoid high-fat, oily, or zesty foods, or those with solid scents. Eat dry foods, like saltines or toast, at regular intervals—taste clear fluids like stocks, sports beverages, and water.

- *Mouth or throat issues:* For sores, agony, or inconvenience gulping, stay with soft foods. Keep away from anything harsh or scratchy and fiery or acidic foods. Eat dinners tepid (not hot or cold). And utilize a straw for soups or beverages.

- *Looseness of the bowels and clogging:* For the runs, it's truly important to remain hydrated. Drink loads of fluids, and cut back on high-fiber foods like whole grains and vegetables. Assuming you're blocked up, gradually add high-fiber foods to your diet. A lot of fluids is key for this issue as well.

- *Change in taste:* Treatment can entertainingly affect your taste buds. Things you could have done without before could taste great at this point. So be open for new foods. Check whether you like acrid or tart flavors, like ginger or pomegranates. Flavors like rosemary, mint, and oregano could assist you with getting a charge out of different foods.

"Cancer Diets"

Many individuals promote "exceptional" diets that they say will assist with treating cancer or keep it from returning. Perhaps you've heard that you ought to go veggie lover, vegan, or begin a crude diet. Before you roll out any major improvements, converse with your doctor.

No diet can fix cancer. Additionally, no decent examination shows that any eating plan, similar to a vegan diet, for instance, can lower the opportunity of cancer returning.

Healthy Mushroom Risotto with Brown Rice

INGREDIENTS

- 6 to 8 cups low sodium vegetable or chicken broth
- 2 teaspoons olive oil
- 1 onion, chopped
- 3 cloves garlic, minced
- 2 (8oz.) containers mushrooms, sliced (I like baby bellas)
- 1/2 teaspoon kosher salt
- 1/2 teaspoon freshly cracked black pepper
- 2 cups brown rice
- 1 cup dry white wine
- 3/4 cup gruyere or good quality parmesan cheese, grated
- 1 teaspoon of "Root Natural Barrier Support"

INSTRUCTIONS

1. In a saucepan, keep the broth warm over low heat.
2. In a large heavy-bottomed pot, heat oil over medium heat. Add onions, garlic, and mushrooms. Sauté until vegetables are soft, about 5 minutes.
3. Add rice, salt, and pepper and cook, stirring, until rice is toasted, about 2 minutes.
4. Add wine and deglaze the bottom of the pan by scraping the browned bits with a spoon. Turn heat down to medium low and stir until liquid is absorbed.
5. Add broth, about half a cup at a time, stirring until liquid is just absorbed each time. Keep adding liquid and stirring until rice is fully cooked and creamy. It will take about an hour to an hour and a half.
6. Once rice is fully cooked and creamy, stir in grated cheese.
7. Serve hot.

NOTES

- It may seem like the rice will never soften. It will. Keep stirring.
- If you run out of broth before the rice has softened all the way, add water to the saucepan to keep warm and use it to continue cooking the rice.
- For vegan, omit the cheese and use vegetable broth.

Loaded Cheesy Potato Soup—Healthy Version

INGREDIENTS

- 4 slices of uncured bacon, chopped
- 1 medium yellow onion, peeled and diced
- 5 cups diced Yukon gold potatoes (from about 5 medium potatoes)
- 3 cloves garlic, peeled and minced
- 1 ½ teaspoons coarse salt
- ½ teaspoon ground black pepper
- ½ teaspoon celery salt
- ½ teaspoon ground mustard
- ⅛ teaspoon cayenne pepper
- ¼ cup all-purpose flour
- 4 cups unsalted vegetable stock
- 1 cup milk
- 1 ½ cups shredded mild or white cheddar cheese
- 1 cup shredded sharp cheddar cheese, divided
- Juice of ½ medium lemon
- 3 medium green onions, thinly sliced (optional)
- 1 teaspoon "Root Restore"

INSTRUCTIONS

1. Heat a Dutch oven or stock pot to medium. Add the chopped bacon and cook 8 to 10 minutes, frequently stirring, until browned and crisp. Use a slotted spoon to transfer it to a paper towel-lined plate.

2. Add the onion to the pot and sauté 4 to 5 minutes, until soft. Add potatoes, reduce heat to low and cook 5 to 7 minutes with the lid on, stirring occasionally. Add the garlic, salt, black pepper, celery salt, ground mustard, and cayenne pepper and sauté 30 to 60 seconds. Stir in the flour.

3. Whisk in the stock and bring to a simmer for about 15 to 20 minutes, until potatoes are soft. Stir in the milk and bring to a simmer, about 3 to 4 minutes, until thickened. Remove from the heat, and stir in the mild or white cheddar cheese and half of the sharp cheddar cheese until melted. Use a potato masher to mash the soup, until about half of the potatoes are mashed. Stir in lemon juice. Taste and adjust seasoning, if necessary.

4. Serve the soup topped with the cooked bacon, the remaining sharp cheddar cheese, and green onion (if using).

NOTES

*Any potato works for this recipe. If you use reds, leave the skin on. If you use russet, peel them first.

Chocolate Quinoa Energy Bars

Serves 12

INGREDIENTS

- ¾ cup unsweetened cocoa powder
- ½ cup whole wheat pastry flour
- ½ cup, plus 2 tablespoons raw shelled hemp seeds, divided
- 1⅓ cups (7.5 ounces) packed pitted dried dates
- 4 large eggs
- ⅔ cup fat free milk or unsweetened plant-based milk
- ½ cup coconut nectar or honey
- 1½ teaspoons pure vanilla extract
- 1 teaspoon sea salt
- ¼ cup grapeseed oil
- ⅓ cup dry quinoa, rinsed and well drained
- 1 teaspoon "Root Relive Greens" * Please see page X for more information on The Root Brands products.

INSTRUCTIONS

1. Preheat the oven to 325°F. Line the bottom of a 9x13-inch nonstick baking pan with parchment paper and set aside. Stir together cocoa powder, flour, and ½ cup hemp seeds in a medium bowl and set aside. Place dates, eggs, milk, coconut nectar, vanilla extract, and salt in a blender. Cover and purèe on high for about 1 minute.

2. Add grapeseed oil and purèe on high for about 30 seconds. Pour contents into a large bowl. Add the cocoa mixture and stir until just combined. Add quinoa and stir until it's evenly combined.

3. Pour batter into the prepared pan. Sprinkle with the remaining 2 tablespoons hemp seeds. Bake until it's springy to the touch, about 35 minutes.

4. Remove from the oven and cut into 12 bars. Cool completely in the pan on a cooling rack, then remove bars. Enjoy at room temperature or chilled from the freezer.

- For flavor variations use different oils, such as peanut, coconut, or walnut oil.

CHAPTER 3

Nutritional Recipes to Support Antiviral Approaches

During flu season or seasons of illness, individuals frequently look for exceptional food varieties or nutrient enhancements that are accepted to help immunity. L-ascorbic acid and food sources like natural citrus products, chicken soup, and tea with honey are well-known models. However, the plan of our immune system is intricate and influenced by an ideal balance of many variables, not simply diet, and particularly not by any one explicit food or supplement. In any case, a decent eating routine comprising a scope of nutrients and minerals, combined with solid life factors like satisfactory rest, exercise, and low stress, prepares the body to battle contamination and sickness.

What Is Our Immune System?

We are consistently presented with possibly harmful microbes. Our immune system, an organization of mind-boggling stages and pathways in the body, safeguards us against these harmful microbes and specific sicknesses. It perceives unfamiliar intruders like microorganisms, infections, and parasites, and makes a quick move. People have two kinds of immunity: intrinsic and versatile.

Intrinsic immunity is the first-line safeguard from microorganisms that attempt to enter our bodies, accomplished through defensive hindrances. These boundaries include:

- Skin that keeps out most microorganisms
- The bodily fluid that traps microbes
- Stomach acid that annihilates microbes
- Chemicals in our sweat and tears that assist with making bacterial mixtures
- Immune system cells that assault all unfamiliar cells entering the body

Versatile or obtained immunity is a system that figures out how to perceive a microbe. It is managed by cells and organs in our body like the spleen, thymus, bone marrow, and lymph nodes. When a foreign substance enters the body, these cells and organs make antibodies and lead to increased immune cells (counting various white platelets) that are intended for that harmful substance, and assault and obliterate it. Our immune system then adjusts by recalling the unknown substance so that, assuming it enters once more, these antibodies and cells are much more effective and fast to obliterate.

Different Circumstances That Trigger an Immune Reaction

Antigens are substances the body marks as unfamiliar and harmful, triggering immune cell movement. Allergens are one kind of antigen and incorporate grass dust, dust, food parts, or pet hair. Antigens can cause a hyper-receptive reaction in which too many white cells are delivered. Individuals' aversion to antigens differs broadly. For instance, a sensitivity to shape triggers side effects of wheezing and hacking in a delicate individual, yet doesn't set off a response in others.

Aggravation is a significant, ordinary move toward the body's intrinsic immune reaction. At the point when microbes assault sound cells and tissue, a kind of immune cell called pole cells counterattack and deliver proteins called receptors, which cause irritation. Irritation might produce suffering, widening, and the appearance of liquids to assist with flushing out the microbes. The receptors additionally convey messages to release much more white platelets to battle microorganisms. Notwithstanding, delayed aggravation can prompt tissue harm and may overpower the immune system.

Autoimmune problems like lupus, rheumatoid joint pain, or Type 1 diabetes are part of the way genetic s can cause touchiness in immune cells and assault and obliterate solid cells.

Immunodeficiency issues can push down or handicap the immune system and might be hereditary or procured. Gained structures are normal and incorporate AIDS and malignant growths like leukemia and numerous myeloma. In these cases, the body's protections are diminished to such an extent that an individual turns out to be exceptionally defenseless to sickness from attacking microorganisms or antigens.

What Elements Can Push Down Our Immune System?

Older age: As we age, our inner organs might become less proficient; immune-related organs like the thymus or bone marrow produce fewer immune cells expected to ward off contaminations. Maturing is sometimes related to micronutrient inadequacies, which might demolish a declining immune capability.

Natural toxins: Smoke and different particles adding to air contamination, these substances can debilitate or stifle the typical movement of immune cells.

Excess weight: Obesity is related to second-rate persistent irritation. Fat tissue produces adipocytokines that can advance incendiary cycles, but the research is early. However, heftiness has likewise been distinguished as a free-risk factor for the influenza infection, conceivably because of the impeded capability of T-cells, a sort of white platelet.

Terrible eating routine: Malnutrition or an eating regimen ailing in at least one supplement can weaken the creation and action of immune cells and antibodies.

Ongoing infections: Autoimmune and immunodeficiency problems assault and possibly impair immune cells.

Persistent mental stress: Stress discharges chemicals like cortisol that smothers aggravation (irritation is at first expected to enact immune cells) and the activity of white platelets.

Absence of rest and sleep: Sleep is a period of rebuilding for the body, during which a sort of cytokine is delivered that battles contamination; too little rest brings down how much these cytokines and other immune cells can fight off contamination or infection.

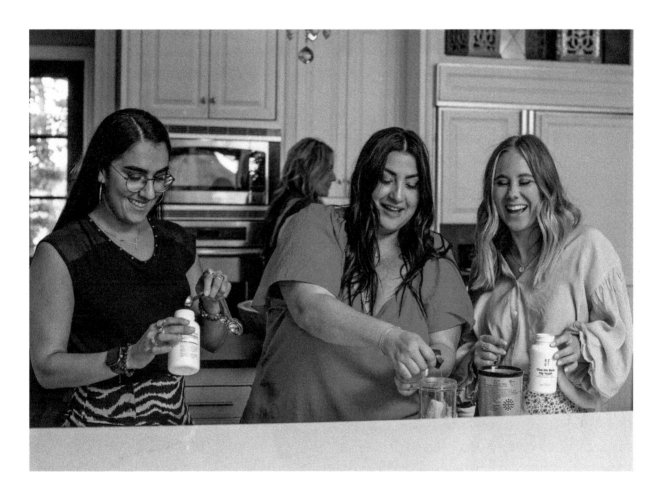

Does an Immune-Boosting Diet Exist?

Eating enough supplements as a feature of a different diet is expected for the well-being and function of all cells, including immune cells. Certain dietary examples might better set up the body for microbial assaults and overabundant inflammation. However, it is far-fetched that singular foods offer exceptional protection. Each phase of the body's immune response depends on the presence of numerous micronutrients. Instances of supplements that have been recognized as the basis for the growth and function of immune cells incorporate

L-ascorbic acid, vitamin D, zinc, selenium, iron, and protein (counting the acid amino glutamine). They are found in various plant and animal foods.

Diets that are restricted in assortment and lower in supplements, for example, consisting of super-processed foods and ailing in negligibly processed foods, can adversely influence a sound immune system. It is also accepted that a Western diet high in refined sugar and red meat and low in soil products can promote aggravations in good gastrointestinal microorganisms, bringing about chronic stomach inflammation and associated smothered immunity.

The microbiome is an inner metropolis of trillions of microorganisms or microbes that live in our bodies, mostly in the digestion tracts. It is an area of extraordinary and dynamic examination, as researchers find that the microbiome is vital in immune function. The stomach is a major site of immune movement and the production of antimicrobial proteins. [6,7] The diet assumes an enormous part in figuring out what sorts of microbes live in our digestive organs. A high-fiber, plant-rich diet with many natural products, vegetables, whole grains, and fruits seem to support the growth and upkeep of gainful microbes. Certain accommodating microbes separate strands into short-chain unsaturated fats, which have been shown to animate immune cell action. These filaments are sometimes called prebiotics because they feed microbes. Therefore, a diet containing probiotic and prebiotic foods might be useful. Probiotic foods contain live, accommodating microbes, and prebiotic foods contain fiber and oligosaccharides that feed and keep up with sound colonies of those microscopic organisms.

Probiotic foods incorporate kefir, yogurt with live dynamic cultures, matured vegetables, sauerkraut, tempeh, kombucha tea, kimchi, and miso. Prebiotic foods incorporate garlic, onions, leeks, asparagus, Jerusalem artichokes, dandelion greens, bananas, and ocean growth. However, a more basic principle is to eat various natural products, vegetables, beans, and whole foods. You're going to eat; why not eat food that can assist you with remaining solid, battling sicknesses, and living longer. You have the power to battle against the infections you are exposed to. There are many tools available, like cleaning up your diet, exercising, and getting a pleasant evening's rest. However, one of the most important ways of avoiding becoming ill is to stay away from eating viral foods. There are a ton of accessible foods to choose from, yet we have gathered the top choices that are not difficult to keep on hand.

Top Anti-Viral Foods

This rundown is comprised of simple foods that you may have in your home. You might not have known how powerful they are, but you should incorporate as many of these into your normal diet as you can, to fend off any infections you are exposed to.

Apple cider vinegar: This enemy of viral food works in two ways. It has every one of the antiviral properties of apples and the probiotics that normally occur when it is aged. A traditional medication now has numerous modern investigations to back up its effectiveness as a microbial specialist. Apple cider vinegar is also perfect for helping digestion too.

Dark tea: Dark tea is an extraordinary enemy of viral food. It contains compounds that battle pathogens—infections, microscopic organisms, and growths. Alkaloids, caffeine, catechins, polyphenols, theobromine, and theophylline are normally occurring components in tea leaves. Studies have shown that dark tea can stop the movement of both influenza and herpes simplex infections. Be careful with the caffeine in dark tea, if you're sensitive.

Green tea: Green tea has a considerable amount of medical advantages over dark tea and has less caffeine. This is a gainful option, on the off chance that you are sensitive to caffeine or in adrenal exhaustion.

Cinnamon: This delicious spice has been utilized restoratively for some years to battle infections, growths, yeasts, microscopic organisms, other microbes, and inflammation. It is also considered an immunomodulator, with its capacity to modify the immune system responses and functions. The smell alone has the potency to stop the growth of certain infections, and it very well may be especially viable with stomach-related bugs.

Garlic: Garlic has been utilized for hundreds of years for its healing properties. It contains extremely strong components that avert a couple of various assortments of herpes, influenza, HIV, pneumonia, and the rotavirus. One of its compounds, allicin, was given to people in a preliminary test for 12 weeks, and it lowered the number and duration of colds compared to a placebo group. So not only is it viable in forestalling colds, but it can also diminish your symptoms on the off chance you get a bug. You might get garlic as an enhancement now.

Ginger: Ginger is old therapeutic food that has been utilized for thousands of years for viral diseases like influenza, the common cold, and human respiratory syncytial infection, or HRSV. One investigation found that it protects cells so the infection cannot append to them while simultaneously starting components to be delivered to battle against the actual infection.

Mushrooms: All edible mushrooms can assist with supporting the immune system. Shiitake mushrooms, specifically, are a powerful enemy of viral foods, and they can hinder the replication of infections, upgrade the immune system, and decrease inflammation. Shiitake mushrooms have strong antifungal and antibacterial components that work against a whopping 85% of the molds and yeasts in the environment.

Yogurt: Yogurt is loaded with probiotics that are perfect for battling infections brought about by contamination, particularly respiratory sicknesses, illnesses that create looseness of the bowels, HIV-1, and specific kinds of Coxsackievirus. If you are in the cutting-edge phases of adrenal exhaustion, be cautious with dairy. Goat yogurt might be a gentler option, or have a go at getting probiotics from other sources.

Oregano: Oregano isn't only an incredible spice for seasoning, it is also hostile to viral properties. Oregano has been found to be compelling against over 30 distinct sorts of organisms, and it's accessible as oil, tea, or supplement.

These are basic, regular foods that are exceptionally simple to incorporate into your diet. They are hostile to viral food and you can eat consistently, to keep you sound and your immune system functioning optimally.

Jamu Juice (Indonesian Turmeric Drink)

INGREDIENTS

- ¾ cup fresh turmeric root (about 100 g), washed and sliced (you may leave the skin intact)*
- 1 large piece of fresh ginger (about 4 inches), washed and sliced (you may leave the skin intact)
- 4 cups water
- 1 pinch freshly ground black pepper
- 2 tablespoons honey
- 2 lemons, juiced
- 1 teaspoon "Root Restore"

DIRECTIONS

1. Place the turmeric, ginger, water, and pepper into a blender. Blend on high until the mixture is completely smooth.
2. Pour the mixture into a medium saucepan and bring to a simmer over medium-high heat. Lower heat and continue simmering for 15 minutes.
3. Once the mixture is done cooking, remove from heat and allow to cool slightly before pouring it through a fine-mesh strainer (or cheesecloth).
4. Add the honey and lemon juice, and serve chilled. The mixture will separate naturally while chilling, so give it a gentle stir before serving.

*Note: If you don't have fresh turmeric on hand, don't worry. Use 1 tablespoon ground turmeric in place of the fresh turmeric root in this recipe and enjoy!

Jicama Daikon Slaw with a Cilantro-Lime Dressing

INGREDIENTS

- ½ jicama, peeled and cut into julienne strips
- 1 daikon radish, cut into julienne strips
- 1 jalapeño, stem and seeds removed, finely chopped (use less if you prefer more mild flavors)
- 3 limes, juiced
- 2 tablespoons rice vinegar
- 2 tablespoons extra virgin olive oil
- 1 clove garlic, minced
- ½ teaspoon kosher salt
- 1 pinch crushed red pepper (optional)
- ¼ cup chopped fresh cilantro

DIRECTIONS

1. Place the jicama, daikon, and jalapeño in a medium mixing bowl.
2. In a separate bowl, whisk together the lime juice, rice vinegar, oil, garlic, salt, red pepper, if using, and cilantro. Pour the dressing over the slaw mixture and gently mix to combine. Serve immediately or refrigerate until ready to enjoy.

Nutrition per serving: 80 calories, 5g total fat, 0.7g saturated fat, 1g protein, 10g carbohydrates, 3.8g fiber, 3g sugar, 0g added sugar, 109mg sodium

Winter Citrus Yogurt Bowl

INGREDIENTS

- 2 cups plain nonfat Greek yogurt
- 1 blood orange, peeled and sliced into rounds
- ¼ cup granola
- 2 tablespoons unsalted pepitas or other nuts or seeds of your choice
- ¼ cup fresh blueberries, rinsed
- 1 tablespoon honey (optional)

DIRECTIONS

1. Divide yogurt into 2 serving bowls. Top each bowl with half of the orange slices, granola, pepitas, and blueberries. Drizzle with honey, if desired.

Nutrition per serving: 305 calories, 6g total fat (1.3g saturated fat), 30g protein, 32g carbohydrates, 3.4g fiber, 20g sugar (3.5g added sugar), 98mg sodium

The Viral Slayer

INGREDIENTS

Broth

- 6 New Mexico chilies
- 2, 2-inch chunks peeled ginger
- 6 shallots, rough chopped
- 4 cloves of garlic
- 2 bunches of cilantro stems
- 1 tablespoon turmeric
- 1 tablespoon fresh thyme
- 1 tablespoon salt
- 2 tablespoons avocado oil
- 1 to 2 pounds ground chicken, depending on how much meat you would like. If you have leftover chicken, you can always use that.
- 3 cups shiitake mushrooms, sliced
- 3 cups maitake mushrooms, broken apart
- 4 cups chicken bone broth. I personally like Bone to Broth, a South Lake Tahoe-based company or Bonafied Provisions, found in the freezer section of the grocery store.
- 1/2 cup apple cider vinegar

Power stash pack, immune-boosting herbs in a tea ball or wrapped in cheesecloth to simmer in broth
- 4 to 5 slices of dried astragalus root
- 3 tablespoons dried nettle leaf
- 1 bunch of kale, sliced
- 1 package of cooked rice noodles; substitute for shirataki or yam noodles if you have Candidiasis, previous head injuries, or ADHD.

Fire paste

- 3 tablespoons fresh ginger, grated
- 2 tablespoons fresh garlic, grated
- 1 to 2 teaspoons cayenne, depending on how spicy you like it
- 2 Meyer lemons, zest only

- 1/3 cup olive oil
- 1 teaspoon salt

Toppings
- Fresh cilantro leaves
- Grated carrots
- Sliced red onions
- Lemon wedges
- Pumpkin seeds
- Sesame seeds
- Fire paste
- Salt

INSTRUCTIONS

Broth

1. Place chilies in a heatproof bowl, add boiling water to cover and let soak until softened, 25 to 30 minutes. Drain chilies, reserving the soaking liquid, remove stems.
2. In a Vitamix or blender, purèe chilies, ginger, shallots, garlic, cilantro stems, turmeric, thyme, and salt.
3. Add 2 cups of the soaking liquid, adding more if needed, until smooth.
4. In a large soup pot, add avocado oil and brown chicken.
5. Add chili mixture to the chicken and cook for 5 minutes, reducing some of the liquid, stirring frequently, making sure not to burn the bottom of the pan.
6. Add mushrooms, broth, apple cider vinegar, power stash pack, and simmer for 30 to 40 minutes.
7. Remove the power stash pack before serving.

Fire paste

1. To make the fire paste, place all the ingredients in a small bowl, stir to combine.

To assemble

1. To assemble the noodles bowls, add cooked rice noodles, ladle hot broth mixture and top with the goodies to make your own personal style.

Orange and Radish Salad with a Citrus Vinaigrette

INGREDIENTS

For the salad:
- 6 cups mixed salad greens
- 1 orange, peeled and sliced into rounds
- 1 radish, thinly sliced
- 2 tablespoons chopped walnuts
- 2 tablespoons goat cheese, crumbled

For the dressing:
- 1 orange, juiced
- 2 tablespoons white wine vinegar
- 1 tablespoon mild olive oil
- ¼ teaspoon kosher salt
- ¼ teaspoon freshly ground black pepper
- 1 teaspoon honey

DIRECTIONS

1. Evenly divide the mixed greens between two serving plates. Top each plate with half of the orange slices, radish slices, walnuts, and cheese.
2. In a small bowl, whisk together the ingredients for the dressing. Pour over the salad just before serving.

Nutrition per serving: 224 calories, 14g total fat (3.2g saturated fat), 6g protein, 21g carbohydrates, 4.4g fiber, 14g sugar (2.9g added sugar), 211mg sodium

Asparagus Antiviral Soup

INGREDIENTS

- 1 14-ounce box of vegetable broth
- 1/4 cup water
- 1 yellow potato, cut into 1/2-inch chunks
- 1 medium shallot, sliced
- 1 clove garlic, minced
- 1/2 teaspoon dried thyme
- 1/2 teaspoon dried marjoram
- 1/8 teaspoon salt
- 12 ounces asparagus (cut off the woody ends and chop into 1-inch chunks)
- Pinch of black pepper
- 1 Teaspoon "Root Natural Barrier Support"

DIRECTIONS

1. In a big pot, boil all the ingredients except for the asparagus. Once boiling, reduce the heat to a simmer and let everything cook until the potatoes are tender. This may take approximately 10 minutes. Once the potatoes are soft, add in the asparagus and cook for another five minutes or until the asparagus is tender.

2. Pour the entire pot of ingredients into a blender and blend until creamy. Enjoy with a sprinkling of black pepper. You can also enjoy this soup chilled the next day or for a refreshing meal on a hot day.

Secret tip: This soup is amazing on its own, but you can also drizzle it over whole-grain brown rice, cubed smoked tofu, or other side dishes to make it a heavier meal.

Nutritional Recipes to Support Bacterial Infection

Your body is comprised of trillions of beneficial bacteria that live on your skin and in your stomach and mucous cells. A few bacteria separate food into absorbable nutrients, synthesize vitamins, obliterate infection-causing cells, and have the insusceptible backing capability, as per the National Academies.

Be that as it may, other microorganisms are liable for contamination. Microorganisms such as viruses, infectious bacteria, and other microbes, can enter your body through your mouth, eyes, nose, or serious injuries. These microorganisms might deliver toxins and can likewise increase and spread throughout your body.

In light of these attacking microorganisms, your body's resistant framework gets a move on. The resistant framework is a mysterious and modern organization of specific cells and tissues, organs, proteins, and synthetics that cooperate to safeguard your body against risky diseases.

An expedient relationship exists between your generally nutritious well-being and the legitimate working of your resilient framework. Your capacity to battle contamination and sickness relies upon your insusceptibility, so it's vital to eat food varieties that battle disease and assist with fortifying your normal safeguards.

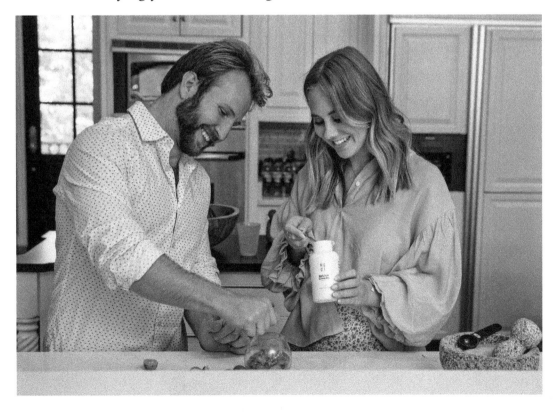

Food Varieties Rich in Antioxidants

Certain vitamins, minerals, and phytonutrients in food support and fortify your safe framework. These are called antioxidants and safeguard your cells from the impacts of free radicals.

Free radicals are particles delivered as side-effects of metabolic cycles, for example, when your body breaks down food, or from natural variables, like exposure to tobacco smoke and radiation.

L-ascorbic acid is a significant physiological cancer prevention agent and may try and assist with recovering other antioxidants in your body, including vitamin E, as per the National Institute of Health. Low degrees of L-ascorbic acid can hinder resistance, and promote higher weakness to contaminations, reports a November 2017 survey in the diary *Nutrients*. As scientists note, this nutrient may forestall and treat respiratory and fundamental contaminations.

Another audit distributed in *Nutrients* in March 2017 noticed that L-ascorbic acid levels in white platelets are multiple times higher than in plasma, which might demonstrate the practical job of the nutrient in resistant capability. Creators report that enormous animal concentrates, that of L-ascorbic acid might help forestall, abbreviate, and reduce various diseases, and propose there is proof that L-ascorbic acid has comparative impacts on people.

This nutrient is known for its relationship with the normal virus. Despite the fact that L-ascorbic acid won't keep you from surrendering to the viral disease of a cold a meta-examination of nine preliminaries, distributed in *BioMed Research International* in July 2018, found that L-ascorbic acid supplementation might abbreviate the span and seriousness of the sickness.

The best L-ascorbic acid food sources, as indicated by the USDA, include:

- Guavas
- Kiwi (organic)
- Strawberries
- Oranges
- Papaya
- Kale

Vitamin E is another one of the normal healing food sources for sicknesses. Its cancer prevention properties can shield your cells from oxidation and subsequently add to keeping issues from contamination. This nutrient may likewise affect respiratory parcel contaminations.

A review distributed in the *European Journal of Clinical Nutrition* in January 2017 surveyed the dietary admission of 1,533 Swedish adults were followed for 9 months and presumed that the admission of vitamin E, as well as L-ascorbic acid, had a backward relationship with the frequency of upper respiratory parcel disease in women.

The top food sources high in vitamin E that can assist with warding off contamination, as revealed by the USDA, are:

- Sunflower seeds and almonds
- Spinach
- Avocados
- Squash
- Kiwifruit
- Trout
- Olive oil

Carotenoids, which incorporate beta-carotene and lycopene, are likewise significant for keeping up with your invulnerable framework. These substances are responsible for the brilliant colors in many foods grown from the ground. Think bright colors while picking strong cancer prevention, agent-rich carotenoid food sources. The USDA records the accompanying food sources as being high in this nutrient:

- Yams
- Carrots
- Dull salad greens
- Butternut squash
- Melon
- Red bell peppers

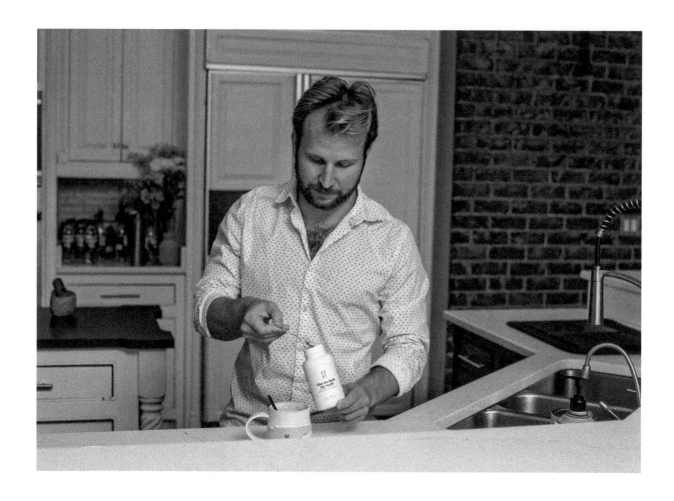

Food Varieties That Support Wound Healing

Numerous food varieties have antimicrobial and antibacterial properties that might assist with accelerating twisted healing by reducing oxygen molecules and inhibiting the reproduction of bacteria that can prompt skin infections.

Garlic is among the food varieties that battle infection and has been utilized medicinally to heal wounds for quite a long time. According to the Linus Pauling Institute, the beneficial effects come from a chemical in garlic called allicin.

Allicin is set free from garlic when you crush or chop it, and it is responsible for garlic's distinct taste and smell. This compound separates to frame an assortment of organosulfur compounds that apply for infection-battling credits, making them normal bacteria executioners.

Zinc likewise has antimicrobial and antibacterial properties that assume a part in injury healing. As well as supporting the safe framework, zinc is a cofactor for some chemicals expected for cell film fix, collagen production, protein union, and cell expansion, which are all fundamental for tissue recovery, according to the National Institutes of Health (NIH).

This mineral assists your skin with remaining solid, and a deficiency might cause skin ulcers and deferred wound healing, which could offer bacteria the chance to attack your tissue and cause infection.

According to the NIH, food varieties that contain zinc might decrease your susceptibility to infection and include:

- Clams
- Red meat and poultry
- Fish
- Fortified breakfast cereals
- Beans
- Nuts
- Entire grains

Antibacterial Herbs and Spices

Many commonly utilized herbs and spices contain antimicrobial and antibacterial compounds that assist with battling infection. Some of these include cloves, oregano, thyme, cinnamon, and cumin. A survey distributed in the *International Journal of Molecular Sciences* (IJMS) in June 2017 summed up the significance of spices relating to their potential use for food safeguarding and treatment of certain infections. These include:

Ginger: Gingerol, which gives ginger its sharp taste, is ginger's critical antifungal and antimicrobial fixing. The audit creators detailed that ginger additionally showed antibacterial activity against every single tried microorganism, including those causing oral infections. Ginger with honey is commonly utilized as a solution for throat congestion and infection.

Cloves: The super active antimicrobial component in cloves is eugenol. Cloves assist with battling infection, as exhibited by their utilization in antiseptics to treat periodontal illness and infection, according to the *IJMS*.

Oregano: The significant antimicrobial components in oregano are carvacrol and thymol. The *IJMS* survey announced these specialists to be effective against a few bacterial infections, such as staphylococcus and salmonella.

Thyme: Thymol is the essential active antimicrobial compound in thyme. The June 2017 *IJMS* survey showed that thyme oil had a high antibacterial effect against 35 bacterial strains tried.

Many individuals have raced to stock up on Emergen- C, elderberry syrup, and vitamin C gummies, trying to help their safe frameworks and keep their family sound.

While you have likely known about inflammation and its connection to serious medical problems like diabetes, joint pain, coronary illness, stroke, and cancer, chances are you haven't investigated what you can change in your eating routine to help your safe framework and battle inflammation.

The resistant framework is answerable for battling unfamiliar trespassers in the body, such as viruses and bacteria, and can likewise obliterate cells inside the body when they become cancerous. Unfortunate sustenance can bring about increased infections, slow healing from injury and infections, and increase susceptibility to side effects and complications from safe framework dysfunction.

What is Inflammation?

Inflammation is your insusceptible framework's reaction to injury, irritation, and infection and is your body's approach to healing cell damage. Chronic inflammation happens when your body goes into overdrive and cannot determine acute inflammation and damage to the body. Lack of exercise, stress, and smoking can set off inflammation. However, dietary choices assume a huge part.

Inflammation can be something you can see, and you can feel it! As a characteristic resistant framework reaction, it assumes a significant part in our capacity to battle infections and keep a solid body. The inflammation that occurs after an injury or cut that causes torment, enlarging, redness, and warmth to the area isn't exactly the issue. It's the other kind of inflammation—the one that is being implicated in pretty much every disease state—the issue lies with that. This kind of inflammation plays a huge part in immune system diseases and contributes significantly to cardiovascular disease and hypertension. It's additionally the main consideration in joint torment and issues like osteoarthritis.

So, how about we check out the various kinds of acute and chronic inflammation so we can all likely understand the difference.

Acute inflammation

Acute inflammation comes on quickly (like inside a couple of moments) and isn't extremely lengthy. This inflammation accompanies torment, redness, expansion, and intensity, generally in light of an injury or infection. This kind of inflammation is significant because it assists the body with warding off forceful microorganisms or bacteria and fixes damaged tissue. You could call this "great inflammation," because it functions to protect you and return the harmed or infected region to a condition of balance. However, another side of inflammation isn't completely ideal and, if not controlled, can be destructive to your well-being. It's welcomed by ways of life factors like smoking and inactivity and can likewise be a side effect of heftiness. It's called chronic inflammation.

Chronic inflammation

Chronic inflammation frequently starts similarly to acute inflammation—the invulnerable framework's approach to fixing an abuse or injury to your body tissues. The issues happen when the inflammation never disappears.

Diagnosing Chronic Inflammation

Chronic or "second rate" inflammation is really difficult to analyze. In spite of the fact that there is a test, you can go to that many refer to as C-reactive protein (CRP) in your blood; it's not unmistakable, so it's anything but a very dependable indicator of inflammation. C-reactive protein is a substance produced by the liver due to inflammation. Doctors frequently utilize this test because research shows high degrees of CRP predict coronary conditions and stroke in women—much more so than having elevated cholesterol. Your doctor may likewise test your white platelet count and sedimentation rate. Each of these three markers in the blood can help decide whether there's inflammation in the body and whether it's improving or worsening after some time.

Overseeing Chronic Inflammation

A nourish program is an excellent initial step to restraining the blaze of chronic inflammation. In this program, you not only eliminate the foods known to cause inflammation (sugar, dairy, gluten, etc.) but also realize which foods you're sensitive to and destroy shrewdly. You eat delicious mitigating foods like salad greens, colorful veggies, nuts, seeds, virgin olive oil, and herbs and spices like turmeric, ginger, and rosemary. You likewise figure out how to reduce pressure by taking care of ones self practices. Supplements that can assist with decreasing inflammation and recuperate the stomach are additionally recommended, such as probiotics and fish oil, which are known to assist with battling inflammation.

Favorable to Inflammatory Foods

Foods that can increase inflammation ought to be restricted or kept away from. Instances of favorable to incendiary foods include refined carbs, profoundly processed packaged foods, excess sugar, red meat, processed meat, and broiled foods. Assuming you have any stomach-related issues or have an immune system disease, grains, beans, eggs, and dairy can likewise be incendiary.

Foods That Battle Inflammation

Nuts: Pecans and almonds are an incredible source of vitamin E, a strong cell reinforcement that is critical to a sound-resistant framework. They are likewise a great source of Omega-3 unsaturated fats, which assume a part in managing your body's inflammatory process and controlling stress connected with inflammation.

Dark salad greens: Broccoli, quite possibly the best vegetable you can add to your plate, is loaded with vitamins A, C, and E, as well as fiber. Spinach and kale are rich in vitamin C, antioxidants, and beta carotene, which might increase the infection-battling capacity of our resistant frameworks.

Berries: Strawberries, blueberries, raspberries, and blackberries are packed with fiber, minerals, vitamins, and a cancer prevention agent called anthocyanins. These compounds reduce inflammation, help resistance, and reduce the risk of coronary illness.

Green tea: Both green and black teas are stacked with flavonoids, a kind of cell reinforcement. Green tea is likewise packed with epigallocatechin gallate (EGCG), another strong cancer prevention agent, and EGCG has been displayed to enhance safe function. Green tea is likewise a decent source of an amino acid called L-theanine, which might support the production of microbe battling compounds in your T cells.

Fish: A wide range of fish contain some omega-3 unsaturated fats. However, salmon, mackerel, and cod are among the best sources because they contain larger amounts of protein and omega-3 unsaturated fats. Omega-3 and Omega-6 unsaturated fats are fundamental for the body's development and improvement. Foods low in omega-3 unsaturated fats are associated with chronic provocative conditions and immune system illness.

Extra virgin olive oil: A staple in the Mediterranean diet, virgin olive oil is rich in monounsaturated fats and contains the cell reinforcement oleocanthal. EVOO has been connected to a reduced risk of coronary illness, brain cancer, and other serious medical issues.

Dark chocolate: In addition to the fact that it is rich and fulfilling, it is packed with antioxidants that reduce inflammation, reducing your risk of illness and prompting better maturing. Dark chocolate contains flavanols that are responsible for their mitigating effects and keeping the coating of your systems stable.

There is no evidence that diet alone can cure chronic or serious ailments. Regular visits to your doctor are important, as preventive care can catch common issues before they cause harm. While adding new, whole foods to your plate is vital to filling your body, it is additionally critical to restrict the consumption of foods that can advance inflammation and stifle the body's safe reaction.

Foods That Cause Inflammation

Trans fats: Known to set off systemic inflammation, trans fats are found in cheap foods, processed snacks, cookies, doughnuts, crackers, margarine, and frozen breakfast products. This includes fried foods like french fries, seared chicken, mozzarella sticks, and egg rolls.

Refined carbohydrates: These products contain white flour, like bread, baked goods, pasta, crackers, and cereal—including white rice and white potatoes. Processed carbohydrates are one of the primary contributors to heftiness and numerous chronic conditions.

MSG: Monosodium glutamate (MSG) is a chemical included in a ton of prepared food we eat. It is a flavor enhancer that is added to Asian foods and soy sauce, yet can likewise be found in fast foods, canned soups, salad dressings, deli meats, and franks. MSG can set off chronic inflammation and affect liver well-being.

Sugar-improved refreshments: Limit your intake of pop, energy drinks, sports beverages, and sweet tea. The sugar in these beverages is one of the main causes of weight gain, diabetes, and an increased chance of coronary illness. Settle on an eating routine rich in colorful, cell reinforcement-rich foods to hold inflammation in check and advance, by and large, overall well-being and healing.

Desserts, cakes, cookies, and soda: They aren't rich in nutrients and they're easy to gorge on, which can prompt weight gain, high glucose levels, and elevated cholesterol (all connected with inflammation). Sugar causes your body to deliver incendiary couriers called cytokines, and pop and other sweet beverages are the principal culprits. Mitigating diet specialists frequently say you should completely cut out added sugars, including agave and honey.

High-fat and processed red meats (like wieners): These have a great deal of saturated fat, which can cause inflammation on the off chance that you eat more than a limited quantity each day.

Margarine, whole milk, and cheese: Again, the issue is saturated fat. All things considered, eat low-fat dairy products, which aren't considered fatty products.

French fries, broiled chicken, and other fried foods: Cooking them in vegetable oil doesn't make them sound. Corn, safflower, and other vegetable oils have omega-6 unsaturated fats. You want some omega-6s, yet assuming you get an excess, you lose the balance between omega-6s and omega-3s in your body and end up with more inflammation.

Coffee creamers, margarine, and whatever else with trans fats: Trans fats (look on the label for "to some degree hydrogenated oils") raise LDL cholesterol, which causes inflammation. There's no protected amount to eat, so stay away.

Wheat, rye, and grain: The focus here is gluten, and it's controversial. Individuals who have celiac disease need to stay away from gluten. In any case, for every other person, the science is strong that entire grains are something worth being thankful for.

Dangers of Chronic Inflammation

Inflammation normally happens in your body. Inflammation protects against poisons, infection, and injury; however, when it happens time after time, it can set off diseases. Specialists connect long-haul (chronic) inflammation to:

- Cancer
- Heart disease
- Diabetes
- Alzheimer's disease
- Depression

You can bring down your chances of chronic inflammation by making changes to what you eat.

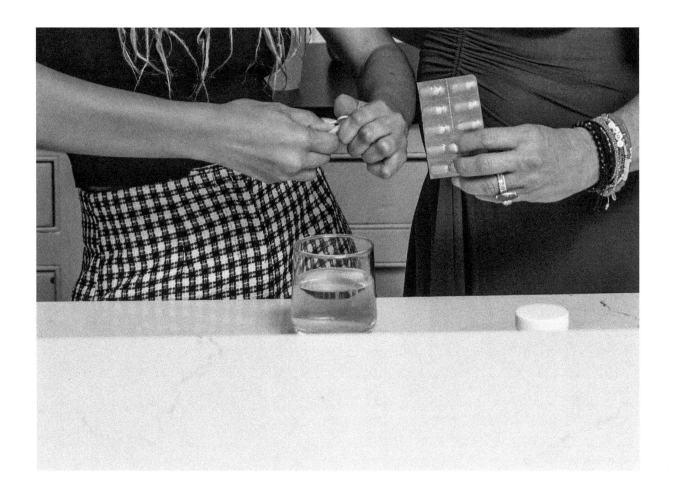

Ginger Turmeric Tea

INGREDIENTS

- 1 tablespoon fresh, grated ginger
- 1 tablespoon fresh, grated turmeric
- 1 whole lemon
- 2 tablespoons maple syrup
- 3 cups water

INSTRUCTIONS

1. Add turmeric, ginger, lemon juice, and leftover lemon rind, maple syrup, and water to a small saucepan.
2. Bring to a simmer over medium to medium-high heat for about 3 minutes and remove from heat.
3. Set a small strainer over two glasses and divide between the two. Enjoy!

Steel Cut Oats with Kefir and Berries

INGREDIENTS

For the oats:

- 1 cup steel cut oats (look for certified gluten-free, if you have a gluten intolerance)
- 3 cups water
- pinch of salt

For topping (these are all optional, and to taste):

- Fresh or frozen fruit/berries (I use blueberries and raspberries, but any fruit will work)
- A handful of sliced almonds, pepitas, hemp seeds, or other nut/seed (you could even use a little of your favorite granola—I'm a fan of Veronica's Health Crunch which is honey & hazelnut granola)
- Unsweetened kefir, homemade or store-bought
- Drizzle of maple syrup, sprinkling of coconut sugar, a few drops of stevia, or any other sweetener you like, to taste

INSTRUCTIONS

1. Add the oats to a small saucepan and place over medium-high heat. Allow to toast, stirring or shaking the pan frequently, for 2 to 3 minutes.
2. Add the water and bring to a boil. Reduce the heat to a simmer, and let cook for about 25 minutes, or until the oats are tender enough for your liking. (The oats will thicken up as they cool—if you prefer them a bit more porridge-like, add a splash more water, or some milk or dairy-free alternative.)
3. Serve with berries, nuts/seeds (or a handful of granola), a splash of kefir, and any sweetener you like, to taste. Dig in!

Chai-Spiced Buckwheat and Chia Seed Porridge

INGREDIENTS

- 1 cup buckwheat, rinsed
- ½ cup oats
- 2 tablespoons chia seeds
- 2 cups milk (cow, almond, or soy)
- 2 cups water
- 1 pear and 1 apple, grated, with skin on
- 1 teaspoon each ground ginger and cinnamon
- ½ teaspoon each ground nutmeg and cardamom
- 2 tablespoons nut butter
- 1 teaspoon vanilla extract
- 2 tablespoons honey

Mixed berry compote

- 500 grams mixed frozen berries
- 1 orange, zest finely grated, and juiced
- ⅓ cup sugar
- 2 teaspoons corn flour
- 1 tablespoon water

METHOD

1. Put the buckwheat and oats in a bowl and cover well with cold water. Put the chia seeds in a separate bowl and add 1 cup of the milk. Leave both bowls on the counter to soak overnight.
2. Drain the buckwheat and oats in a fine sieve, then rinse well under cold water.
3. Place the chia seeds with the milk in a medium saucepan along with the remaining 1 cup milk, the buckwheat and oats, water, grated pear and apple, all the spices, nut butter, vanilla and honey. Cook over a low heat for about 30 minutes, stirring often until thick and creamy, adding more water or milk to keep it at a soft consistency. Serve in bowls topped with your choice of toppings.

COOK'S TIP: The porridge keeps well in the fridge for 5 days. Just heat each serving when needed, adding a little extra liquid if needed.

Gluten-Free Buckwheat Pancakes with Blueberries

INGREDIENTS

- 1 large egg, room temperature
- 1 1/4 cups buttermilk
- 1/4 cup Chobani plain, non-fat yogurt
- 2 tablespoons brown sugar
- 1 tablespoon olive oil
- 1/2 teaspoon vanilla extract
- 1 cup plus 2 tablespoons buckwheat flour
- 1 1/2 teaspoons baking powder
- 1/4 teaspoon cinnamon
- 1/2 teaspoon salt
- 2 cups fresh blueberries
- 1 teaspoon Root Relive Greens

INSTRUCTIONS

1. Heat a large skillet or griddle on medium heat.

2. In a medium bowl combine egg, buttermilk, yogurt, brown sugar, olive oil, and vanilla extract, whisking until combined. In a separate bowl, whisk together buckwheat flour, baking powder, cinnamon, and salt. Incorporate into wet ingredients, stirring only until combined.

3. Once griddle is hot, grease with oil. Pour ¼ cup of batter per pancake onto surface, then sprinkle with blueberries. Cook on one side until holes form around edges, about 1 minute, then flip and cook on other side for additional minutes. Don't let the pan get too hot—you want a nice, even heat.

4. Serve with whipped cream, blueberries, nuts, and a healthy drizzle of maple syrup!

CHAPTER 5

Nutritional Recipes to Support Parasitic Cleanse Diet

If you suspect you might have a parasitic disease, there is a usual method for treating it. It's known as parasite cleansing. Parasitic diseases have become more common with global travel over the long haul. We currently realize that different parasites can contaminate the digestive system, prompting various stomach-related side effects, like constipation, diarrhea, vomiting, and heartburn, as well as fatigue and anxieties.

A parasite cleansing includes eating a diet free from foods that feed parasites (like sugar and grains) and devouring more foods that are hostile to parasites, such as cell reinforcement-rich foods. It's very near a Paleo diet, which furnishes you with fundamental supplements from things like probiotic foods, herbs, vegetables, and more.

Enhancements can likewise be useful for supporting your gastrointestinal and invulnerable frameworks while you recuperate on a parasite purge.

What Are Parasites?

A parasite is an organism that lives on or in a host and gets its food from or to the detriment of its host. The parasite utilizes the assets of the individual it's living within, for example, feeding off the same food that the host eats, to make due. Indeed, it's not lovely.

More terrible, parasites can cause sickness in people. Some infections brought about by these organisms are handily treated, while some are not.

There are three main classes of parasites that can cause illness in people: protozoa, helminths, and ectoparasites. Instances of a few serious parasitic illnesses incorporate filariasis, malaria, and babesiosis.

How Can Somebody Become Tainted with a Parasite?

In all honesty, a generally high level of adults living in the United States might convey parasites. Where and how can someone get contaminated with a parasite?

For the most part, parasites are procured from drinking tainted food or water. Yet, individuals with imbalanced stomach bacteria, a flawed stomach disorder, or a debilitated safe framework might be more powerless. Some can likewise be spread through the chomp of a mosquito or sand fly or communicated to people from animals, for example, cows and pigs that are contaminated with parasites like Cryptosporidium or Trichinella.

One common reason for parasites is eating pork, particularly if it's undercooked or crude. Pork can convey parasites and worms because of the unfortunate circumstances that pigs/swine are ordinarily brought up in, so assuming this kind of meat is consistently remembered for your diet, you might be helpless to convey one.

Different sorts of undercooked meat and seafood can move unsafe organisms, including hamburgers, shellfish, and crab.

Global travel is another expected reason. Assuming that you live in the United States or Europe, yet have at any point been to another nation like China, India, Africa, or Mexico, quite possibly drinking the neighborhood water and eating the food in these spots might have made you get a parasite.

As per the Centers for Disease Control and Prevention (CDC), "Worldwide, polluted water is a difficult issue that can cause extreme torment, inability, and even demise." Contaminated water incorporates drinking water. However, water from pools, hot tubs, lakes, streams, or the sea can also be contaminated.

Assuming you've at any point gotten back from an private excursion and had loose bowels or another stomach-related issue, you may be managing what the CDC calls relentless explorers' diarrhea, which alludes to gastrointestinal side effects that keep going for over 14 days. Per the CDC, the pathogenesis of tireless diarrhea in returned voyagers is sometimes brought about by disease because of a parasitic organism.

As well as being cautious about the food and water you drink while voyaging, legitimate disinfection and cleanliness are likewise fundamental to forestalling parasites and comparative diseases.

Parasite Cleanse Diet

Assuming that you've laid out that you have a parasite, you're likely searching for the best parasite purge to assist you with recuperating. Some portion of the healing system follows a parasite purify diet, while another significant part is enhanced with natural homemade cures.

Below are ideas for following a parasite purge diet as well as additional down-to-earth tips and supplement proposals that can assist with eliminating the worms and parasites in your framework.

1. Parasite Cleanse Supplements

While enhancing to kill parasites, there are natural enemies of parasite intensifies you'll need to utilize. One such item is called ParaComplete, which is a parasite scrub enhancement that contains thyme leaf, something many refer to as berberine sulfate (that you can here and there find in coconut and can kill off parasites), oregano, grapefruit seed extract and uva ursi leaf.

You can likewise make your own parasite purge creation utilizing supplements you can get in color structure. These incorporate dark pecan, wormwood, olive leaf, and garlic.

Intermittently, you can find a parasite scrub with these natural ingredients at your nearby health-food store or get them independently.

Here are the top natural enhancements for your own personal parasite purge:

- Dark pecan (250 milligrams 3x a day, every day)—Has been utilized generally for the treatment of parasites.
- Wormwood (200 milligrams 3x a day, every day)—It's known as an enemy of parasitic properties.
- Oregano oil (500 milligrams 4x a day, every day —Oregano oil has both antibacterial and parasitic impacts.
- Grapefruit seed extract (taken as coordinated)—Has been displayed to have antimicrobial properties against a large number of organisms.
- Clove oil (500 milligrams 4x a day, every day or 4 cups of tea)—Contains high measures of eugenol, a compound that has been displayed to assist with killing hurtful organisms.
- Probiotics (1 or 2 containers every day)—These "hero" microorganisms help repopulate the stomach with organisms that help stomach-related well-being.

Notwithstanding those above, different enhancements that might be useful include:

- anise
- barberry
- berberine
- mint
- goldthread

Most specialists suggest you do around two weeks of a parasite scrub, taking the enhancements above, then go home for the week. After your one-week break, hop into the arrangement again for two additional weeks.

The actual convention is a significant piece of your treatment, similarly as much as taking the supplements. Attempt to stick to the planning of the arrangement to obtain the best outcomes.

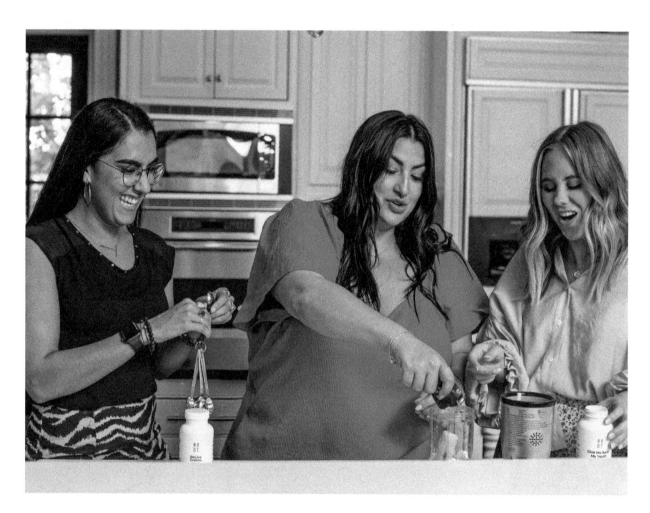

2. Following an Anti-Parasite Diet

A parasite-purge diet helps eliminate hurtful organisms living in your stomach-related framework by battling terrible microorganisms and growth that these parasites live off of. This kind of purification includes following a diet free from all sugar and grains—very near a Paleo diet.

I suggest you limit your natural product admission or eat no organic product. So as opposed to a berry smoothie, drink a coconut smoothie with coconut milk, chia seeds, and protein powder.

For lunch, do a major serving of mixed greens. For supper, prepare natural meat and twofold the vegetables, remaining totally away from any type of grains or sugar, including natural products.

Another food that can be extremely recuperating while battling hurtful organisms in your GI system is pumpkin seeds and pumpkin seed oil. Pumpkin seeds support gastrointestinal health since they contain specific antioxidants and other defensive mixtures, such as tetracyclic triterpenes and cucurbits, which can paralyze worms and make it challenging for them to get by in the digestive barriers.

Eat about one cup of pumpkin seeds a day—for instance, by adding some to a smoothie in the first part of the day, and one more portion of a cup in the early evening, or you can make pumpkin seed spread, tossing this into something like a blender alongside pumpkin seed oil, that most health-food stores ought to carry.

While going through a parasite detox purge, it is critical to help our natural parasite detox tonic with a legitimate anti-parasite diet. Numerous resources are accessible on the most proficient method to dispose of parasites with herbs. However, not as many individuals examine what to eat while consuming these anti-parasitic herbs—and what you eat has a major effect.

Truly, there is no widespread diet for everybody, as diet differs with age, way of life, climate, sensitivities, genetic history, and countless variables. Subsequently, we won't say precisely what to eat in an anti-parasite diet. Instead, we will share the most gainful dietary tips and dinner plan models you can consider while doing a parasite diet and parasite cleanse. We'll likewise incorporate some parasite-cleanse diet recipes. Remember that these are not strict principles, and you want to utilize your judgment in light of your own dietary inclinations while following the anti-parasite diet. The primary concentration for an anti-parasite diet is including anti-parasitic foods and staying away from foods that add to a parasitic climate. It is vital to stay away from specific negative food propensities (like gorging) as a piece of an anti-parasites diet.

How Do You Follow the Parasite-Detox Diet?

To follow the parasite-detox diet, the main thing to do is stick to these standards planned to assist with supporting the disposal of parasites.

Eat Anti-Parasitic Foods

The main tip to follow on a parasite-detox diet is to incorporate anti-parasitic foods for your dinners. These foods have anti-parasitic properties and can assist with taking out parasites from your body. Preferably, you will incorporate at least one of these foods for every one of your dinners:

- garlic
- onion
- honey
- pumpkin seeds
- dates
- pomegranate
- papaya seeds
- dandelion greens
- lettuce
- broccoli
- kale
- pineapple
- coconut
- carrots
- sunflower seeds
- stone-ground mustard
- coconut Oil
- apple cider vinegar
- turmeric
- ginger
- cinnamon
- cayenne Pepper
- curry flavors
- cloves
- thyme
- oregano
- neem

While doing a parasite cleanse, you should incorporate a greater amount of the foods from this list that you, for the most part, would eat. This will assist with supporting the successful detoxification and end of digestive parasites, given that different parts of the diet and convention are additionally adhered to.

Stay Away from Added Sugars

Quite possibly, the main thing to do while following a parasite-detox diet is to keep away from all added sugars. Numerous microorganisms, including different kinds of parasites, feed on sugar as an essential wellspring of energy. Keeping your sugar consumption low, at any rate, can assist with starving these organisms and debilitate them, making them more defenseless against anti-parasitic herbs and foods.

Added sugars are in numerous foods, and we frequently devour them without acknowledging them. Along these lines, it is fundamental that you read the labels on foods and actually look at the ingredients for added sugar. A few normal foods that frequently have added sugar include:

- pop
- caffeinated drinks
- sports drinks
- sauces
- condiments
- salad dressings
- juices
- bottled teas
- cereals
- yeast bread
- candy
- grain-based pastries
- dairy pastries
- syrups
- garnishes
- processed foods

If you are following a parasite-detox diet, it is ideal to focus on real foods in their regular structure, and keep away from added sugars. We prescribe restricting your sugar intake to the morning, when you can eat a modest quantity of low glycemic organic natural products.

When the parasitic contamination is gone, the organic product can be an exceptionally sound piece of a nutritious diet. Notwithstanding, it is prescribed to restrict natural product intake on the parasite-detox diet to keep the parasites from their significant fuel source. We suggest keeping away from stevia, xylitol, erythritol, and different sugars while on the parasite-detox diet.

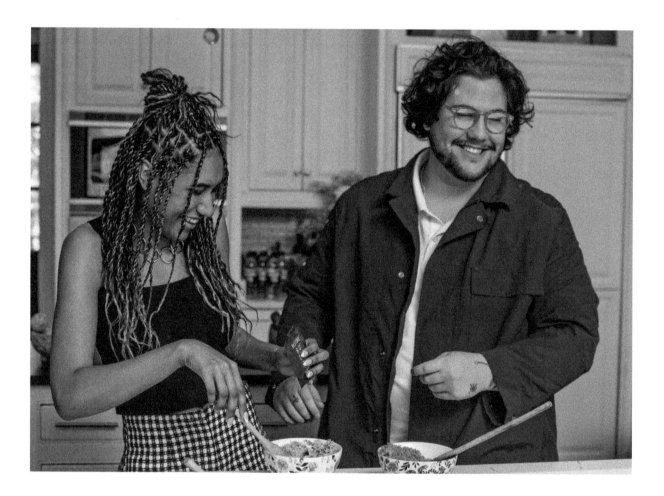

Make a Point to Consume Plenty of Fiber

Eating fiber-rich foods during your parasite cleanse is critical, as these truly assist with cleaning out the gut. Fiber gives the colon the oil it needs to work appropriately and assists with supporting a normal and smooth end. Fiber falls into two classes: soluble and insoluble. Dissolvable (soluble) fiber serves many capabilities, including giving a helpful climate to well-disposed microorganisms, slowing the retention rate of sugars, lowering serum cholesterol levels, and restricting weighty metals unloaded by the circulatory system into the colon. Soluble fiber foods include apples, prunes, figs, raspberries, carrots, oat wheat, kidney beans, lima beans, or (supplemental) psyllium husks.

Insoluble fiber supplements solvent fiber by expanding mass in the waste, forestalling affected gut pockets (diverticula), decreasing the timeframe waste stays in the body, and engrossing bile acid delivered during assimilation. Instances of insoluble fiber are brown rice, quinoa, millet rice, entire wheat, wild spinach, Brussels sprouts, and flaxseed.

Foods that are normally high in fiber:

- Chia seeds
- Chickpeas
- Figs
- Prunes
- Psyllium husks
- Beans
- Broccoli
- Flaxseed
- Berries
- Lentils
- Avocados
- Entire grains
- Apples
- Carrots
- Brown rice
- Wheat grain
- Cereal
- Pears
- Bananas
- Beets
- Artichokes
- Brussels sprouts
- Quinoa
- Popcorn
- Almonds
- Yams

Eat Low-Starch Vegetables

While vegetables are a fundamental nutrition class for any sound diet, including the parasite-detox diet, attempt to limit bland vegetables while following this diet.

Instances of high-starch vegetables to lessen during this diet include:

- white potatoes
- sweet potatoes
- yams
- corn
- peas
- beans

You don't need to totally eliminate these vegetables from your diet. Nonetheless, don't eat such a large number of them and favor, for the most part, green, low-starch vegetables. Center around eating supplements and vegetables that have lower calories.

Here are a few instances of low-starch vegetables to incorporate into your diet during this cleanse:

- spinach
- dandelion greens
- kale
- cherry tomatoes
- ringer peppers
- zucchini
- cucumber
- cauliflower
- Brussels sprouts
- broccoli

While looking for these vegetables, purchase organic and cook them with great oils! Terrible oils can make any good feast into an incendiary bad dream; for more data on the most proficient method to find good cooking oils, read Harvard Health's blog on expanding your healthy cooking oil choices.

Eat Fruits That Are Low In Sugar

While it is prescribed to avoid fruits that are high in sugar, it is alright to incorporate some low-sugar fruits into the diet. As a matter of fact, some low-sugar fruits like lemons, limes, and coconuts contain strong anti-parasitic properties.

It is prescribed to eliminate these high-sugar fruits from the diet altogether during your multi-day parasite cleanse:

- bananas
- mangos
- melon
- grapes
- figs

These fruits can be incorporated during your cleanse day to day:

- limes
- Lemon
- coconut
- pineapple (has strong anti-parasitic properties)
- papaya seeds (have strong anti-parasitic properties)
- pomegranate
- avocados

These fruits should be eaten in moderation, in the morning before any proteins:

- blueberries
- raspberries
- strawberries
- blackberries
- cherries
- apples
- dates (while dates are high in natural sugar, they also contain anti-parasitic properties)

We suggest eating before a protein since protein demands an investment to process, which straightforward sugars can make more troublesome. Toward the beginning of the day, you are in an abstained state, which is great for consuming straightforward sugars.

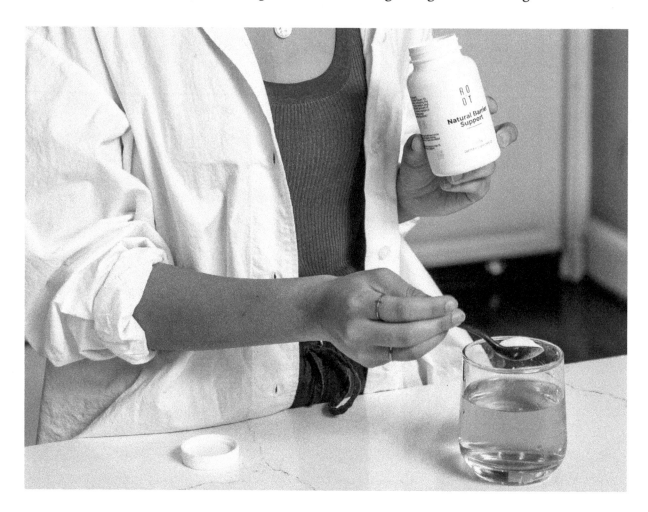

Remember Prebiotic Foods for Your Diet

Prebiotic foods are unpalatable carbs that assist with taking care of useful microscopic organisms in the gastrointestinal tract. Prebiotic foods are extremely advantageous for stomach well-being. While some prebiotic foods contain sugar, the list below contains good prebiotic sources that are low in sugar.

Here are some other top anti-parasite foods:

Garlic and onions: These insusceptible supporting vegetables have anti-parasitic impacts because of their sulfur mixtures and antioxidants that can obliterate pathogenic organisms.

Herbs: Certain herbs, similar to oregano and ginger, can have antibacterial and antiparasitic impacts, since they assist with expanding the creation of stomach acid, which can kill parasites and forestall infections.

Pineapple, papaya, and their juices: These fruits contain intensities that can assist with diminishing the creation of supportive provocative cytokines that can bring about colon aggravation. Their juices can likewise make anti-parasitic impacts.

Coconut oil: Coconut oil has antibacterial and antimicrobial properties.

Probiotic-rich foods: Consuming high-probiotic foods like kefir, sauerkraut, and yogurt can control parasites and improve the stomach's well-being.

Apple cider vinegar: Helps reestablish solid pH balance and can, by and large, improve digestion.

Other new vegetables: These are rich wellsprings of defensive mixtures that assist with feeding the stomach and give fiber, energizing normal solid discharges.

Here are the foods you need to keep away from:

Added sugar: This can take care of dangerous organisms in the stomach and add to aggravation.

Alcohol: Does not allow for appropriate insusceptible framework functioning.

Wheat: Many grains, particularly those containing gluten, can separate into sugar rapidly and cause digestive irritation.

Pork: Can possibly be polluted with parasites.

It's critical to forestall constipation and energize ordinary solid discharges while cleansing, since this frees your body from parasites. A few specialists prescribe doing a couple of colonics to work on gastrointestinal well-being; ordinarily, a few colon cleanses once weekly, for a considerable time. This should be possible while doing the two-to-four-week parasite cleanse.

Together these techniques can be a powerful system for assisting with freeing your group of unsafe organisms while likewise sustaining yourself from the back to front.

Symptoms of parasitic infection:

What are a few signs that you might have a parasite? The most widely recognized side effects of parasitic contamination include:

- Stomach-related issues, including constipation, diarrhea, vomiting, gas, heartburn
- Stomach pains and weakness
- Loss of hunger
- Tiredness

- Chills
- A throbbing painfulness·
- Side effects of dehydration

Here is a rundown of 6 anti-parasitic foods that can assist you with killing parasites normally:

Pineapple: The center of the pineapple is bountiful in a protein known as bromelain, which can support digestion and kill parasites. Pineapple juice can diminish the development of pro-inflammatory cytokines that can bring about colon aggravation.

Bromelain is likewise perfect for separating protein foods, making it extraordinary for battling gastrointestinal parasites, as it can kill worms. Ordinary utilization of pineapple can improve your insusceptible framework and assist it with battling and wiping out parasites.

Pumpkin seeds: Pumpkin seeds are regularly used to regard parasites, as they contain tetracyclic triterpenes, which can assist with eliminating parasites from the body.

Aside from that, pumpkin seeds contain cucurbits that can incapacitate worms and make it hard for them to conceal inside the digestive walls. This works with their expulsion from the body during a solid discharge.

Cucumber seeds: Cucumber seeds are perfect for eliminating tapeworms that dwell in the gastrointestinal system. That is why it is smart to consume cucumber seeds, regardless of whether you have a parasite, as a careful step. The catalysts found in cucumber can kill tapeworms.

However, if you are encountering tapeworms, it is ideal to go straight to an average proficient, like the best gastroenterologist in Karachi.

Garlic: The therapeutic properties of garlic have been known since old times, and it is utilized by individuals all around the world to support craving, reinforce the resistant framework, kill parasites, and treat motion-induced nausea. Garlic is wealthy in sulfur intensifies that can annihilate pathogenic organisms and decline the arrangement of blood clusters.

Garlic can support the creation of stomach acids, which is significant, as constantly low stomach acid has been connected to microorganisms and yeast excess in the stomach.

Ginger: Like garlic, ginger can likewise build the development of stomach acid, which can kill parasites and forestall infections. Aside from that, ginger can increment blood course and is great for a wide range of stomach-related issues.

Apple cider vinegar: Since apple cider vinegar contains B vitamins, it is exceptionally sustaining for the body. It can reestablish normal pH balance, improve digestion, and kill parasites.

Intestinal Parasite-Cleansing Soup

INGREDIENTS

- 1/4 teaspoon clove powder
- 1/4 teaspoon nutmeg powder
- 1/4 black cumin (Nigella seeds) or regular cumin seeds
- 1/4 teaspoon fennel seeds
- 1/4 teaspoon turmeric powder
- 1/4 teaspoon Aijwan seeds
- Black pepper
- Rock salt
- 2 to 3 garlic cloves
- 1 inch fresh ginger
- 2 large leeks
- 3 handfuls of green leaves of your choice
- Pumpkin seeds, for the garnish
- 1 teaspoon coconut oil
- 2 drops "Root Clean Slate"

INSTRUCTIONS

1. Thoroughly wash and chop the veggies.
2. Peel and cut the onion, garlic, and ginger.
3. Heat a little coconut oil in an cast-iron pot.
4. Sauté the onions until soft and fragrant but not too dark.
5. Add the spice seeds and roast them for 1 minute, keeping an eye, so they do not burn.
6. Add the leeks and sauté for 2 to 3 minutes.
7. Add green leaves and boiling water, just enough to cover the veggies.
8. Bring to a boil.
9. Stir in the spice powders.
10. Lower the heat, boil for about 10 to 15 minutes.
11. Add the ginger and garlic (if this is too strong for you i.e. you have a sensitive stomach, you can add the ginger and garlic right after you've sautéed the onion—although it will be less efficient in terms of killing intestinal parasites and worms)

12. Blend with a hand mixer, adding or removing water to reach the desired consistency (and according to your constitution).

13. Add salt and pepper to taste.

14. Garnish with pumpkin seeds.

15. Serve warm! Bon appétit!

Apple Cider Vinegar Parasite-Cleanse Salad Dressing

INGREDIENTS

- 1 to 2 tablespoons raw unfiltered apple cider vinegar
- 4 tablespoons olive oil, unrefined cold pressed extra virgin
- 1 medium lemon
- 2 cloves raw garlic
- ¼ teaspoon Himalayan salt, to taste
- ¼ teaspoon ground black pepper, optional
- ½ teaspoon mustard, optional
- ¼ teaspoon turmeric powder, optional
- 1 teaspoon raw local honey or stevia, optional

INSTRUCTIONS

1. Shake the apple cider vinegar bottle to mix the cloudy part at the bottom (the "mother").
2. In a glass bottle or a mason jar, place 1 to 2 tablespoons of apple cider vinegar.
3. Squeeze the juice of 1 lemon and add to the bottle.
4. Add 4 tablespoons of olive oil. Shake the bottle.
5. Mince the garlic, add to the bottle, and shake well.
6. To make the healthy lemon vinaigrette version, add ½ teaspoon of mustard.
7. Add Himalayan salt and black pepper to taste. Shake well.
8. If you like turmeric, add ¼ teaspoon of ground turmeric and shake well. To add a little sweetness to balance the turmeric flavor, add a few drops of stevia.
9. Add to your salad. Enjoy!

Nutrition—calories: 240kcal

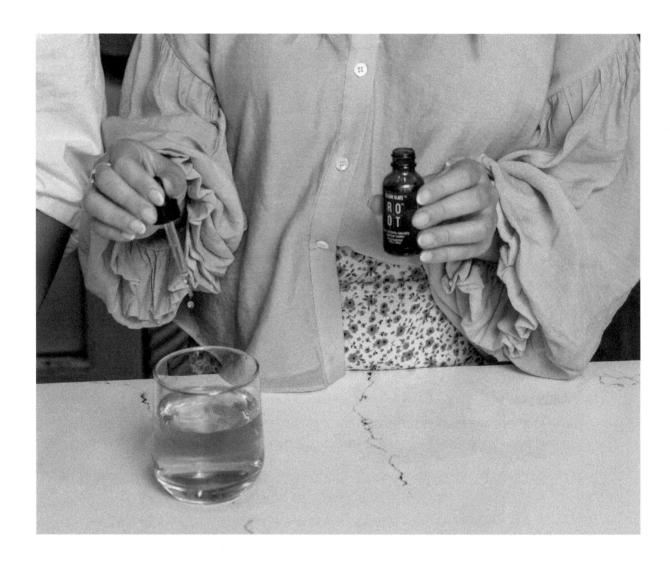

Apple Cider Vinegar Parasite Cleanse

INGREDIENTS

- 16 ounces distilled or spring water, room temperature
- 1 teaspoon raw, unfiltered apple cider vinegar
- 1 small lemon or lime
- 1 teaspoon raw local honey or stevia, optional

INSTRUCTIONS

1. Shake the apple cider vinegar bottle to mix the cloudy part at the bottom (the "mother").
2. Add 1 teaspoon of apple cider vinegar to the 16 ounces of distilled or spring water.
3. Squeeze the juice of 1 organic lemon or lime and add to the drink.

4. For added sweetness, mix a few drops of stevia or 1 teaspoon of raw local honey into the mixture. When using honey, shake the drink.

5. Drink on an empty stomach in the morning, during the day, and before bedtime, up to three times per day, at least 2 hours before or after other meals.

Nutrition—calories: 20kcal

Colon Cleanse Recipe: The Detox Salad Your Gut Will Love

INGREDIENTS

- 1 medium head raw cabbage
- 3 medium raw carrots
- 1 small raw beetroot
- 2 cloves raw garlic
- 1 to 2 small hot cayenne peppers, optional
- 1 to 2 tablespoons raw apple cider vinegar unpasteurized, with the "mother."
- 1 small lemon
- 4 tablespoons olive oil, unrefined cold pressed extra virgin
- 2 oz. raw hemp seeds
- Pink Himalayan salt, to taste

INSTRUCTIONS

1. Peel the beetroot.
2. Shred the cabbage, carrots, and beets. Place in a large bowl.
3. Add minced garlic.
4. Cut the hot peppers into small pieces. This is optional, for people who dislike spicy food.
5. Squeeze the juice of 1 lemon and add to the bowl.
6. Shake the apple cider vinegar bottle to mix the cloudy part at the bottom (the "mother"). Add organic, raw unfiltered unpasteurized apple cider vinegar.
7. Add the olive oil and mix well.
8. Add the salt to balance the flavor.
9. Add the hemp seeds and mix.

NOTES

If possible, try to use as many organic and local ingredients as you can.

Nutrition—calories: 575kcal

Cauliflower Rice Detox Recipe

INGREDIENTS

- 1 head cauliflower
- 1 medium red onion
- 2 to 4 small cayenne peppers, optional
- 2 to 4 cloves garlic
- 2 medium red bell peppers
- 2 medium carrots
- 1 to 2 stalks scallions, optional
- 2 oz. hemp seeds
- 2 oz. unroasted, unsalted almonds
- 2 tablespoons coconut oil, extra virgin raw
- Himalayan pink salt, to taste
- ½ to 1 teaspoon chipotle chili powder, optional
- 1 teaspoon ground turmeric powder, optional
- 1 oz. unfortified nutritional yeast, not for candida diet

INSTRUCTIONS

1. Cut the cauliflower into florets. Remove the stem.
2. Grate the cauliflower florets to get rice-grain size pieces. You can use a food processor or a box grater with medium-size holes.
3. Using paper towels, press the grated cauliflower to remove excess moisture.
4. Chop the red onion, garlic, carrots, scallions (if using), and peppers.
5. Heat the coconut oil in a wok or cast-iron skillet on medium-high heat.
6. Add the chopped red onions and garlic. Sauté until onions turn a light brown color, about 2 to 3 minutes.
7. Add the grated cauliflower and mix well, for 2 to 3 minutes.
8. Add the rest of the veggies and mix well.
9. Taste and add the chipotle chili and turmeric powder, if using, and mix well. Add Himalayan pink salt, as needed.
10. Do not overcook the cauliflower. Keep stirring until all liquids are absorbed and it has your desired consistency.
11. Remove from heat.
12. Right before serving, add the hemp seeds, almonds, and nutritional yeast. Mix well. Enjoy! The nutritional yeast is not recommended for the first few weeks of the candida diet.

CHAPTER 6

Nutritional Recipes to Support Fungal Overgrowth

Fungal overgrowth takes place in humid and warm climatic conditions. It grows when your skin starts getting damaged. Also referred to as yeast, fungal overgrowth usually occurs on the skin, digestive system, and vaginal area among women and around the penis in men. When too much yeast develops in different areas of your skin, it leads to an infection. The infection is also referred to as candidiasis.

It also develops when you have a weak immune system and take antibiotics for the treatment of a specific disease. Antibiotics, especially, are known for killing the healthy bacteria that normally protect your body and keep the growth of yeast in check. Here is a list representing those who are more likely to develop a yeast infection:

- Patients undergoing cancer treatment
- People who take antibiotics
- Infants
- Those wearing dentures
- People suffering from either diabetes or HIV

The most likely places where yeast infection can grow include the mouth, nail beds, around the navel area, penis, and vagina. Some of the most common symptoms related to yeast infection consist of:

- Breakdown of skin
- Burning or itching
- Pimples
- Itchiness, redness, and rashes
- Discharge of white or yellow fluid from the vagina
- Redness around external areas surrounding the vagina
- Redness under the penis
- Difficulty swallowing food, if the infection is in the mouth
- Swelling of the nails
- The white or yellow color of the nails separates them from their beds

If you experience any of the above symptoms, see your doctor immediately for an appropriate diagnosis. Before examining your condition, your healthcare provider will ask you about your medical history and if you have ever experienced similar symptoms before. After inquiring about your medical history, your doctor will physically examine you. They will scrape a small piece of your skin or nail to confirm that you have a yeast infection.

Once an appropriate diagnosis has been made, your doctor will start the required treatment as per your overall health condition, your age, and other essential aspects to determine the type of treatment you may require. Most yeast infections can easily be treated by using anti-fungal creams. The line of treatment is also determined by the location where the infection has started.

For example, to treat yeast infection around the genital areas of males and females, doctors prescribe anti-yeast ointments or medicines. If the infection is in the mouth, a healthcare expert may prefer prescribing medicated mouthwash or lozenges that easily dissolve in your mouth.

As far as esophageal fungal infections are concerned, treatment usually involves intravenous anti-fungal medicines or oral medication.

Similarly, yeast infection located in the nails is also treated with oral anti-fungal medication. Finally, yeast infections of the skin folds are usually treated using anti-yeast powders. If you are wondering how you can prevent yourself from getting a yeast infection, consider the following remedies:

- To prevent getting a yeast infection in your mouth, consider flossing and brushing your teeth using mouthwash on a daily basis. Practice other oral hygiene methods for the same.
- Preventing yeast infection around the vaginal area requires wearing cotton underwear. You can also take probiotics to avoid getting a yeast infection.
- Make sure that the areas of your body where there is friction due to regular skin contact remain dry.

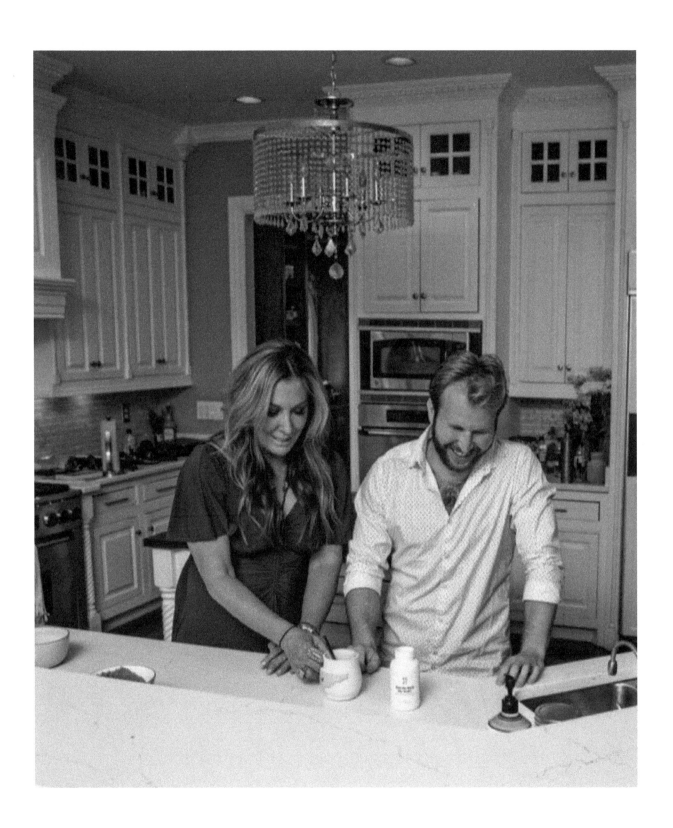

Moreover, your diet and nutrition also play a significant role in helping you prevent or cleanse candida—yeast infections. Some of the most recommended foods in this regard include vegetables and fruits. For example, Brussels sprouts, cabbage, cauliflower, and broccoli. Leafy greens like lettuces, kale, and dandelion. Among less starchy veggies, you can opt for shallots, onions, zucchini, and asparagus. In addition, you can also include turmeric, cumin, ginger, lemon, and some types of fruits. Some of the best fruits to help cleanse candida are blueberries, raspberries, strawberries, and tomatoes.

As far as nuts, seeds, and herbs are concerned, you can eat macadamia nuts, almonds, walnuts, chia seeds, hemp seeds, flaxseed, cilantro, oregano, and basil. Among other edibles you can rely on to get rid of candida, go for dark chocolate, water, green tea, bone broth, coconut oil, avocado, olives, olive oil, and rooibos.

Make sure that you completely eliminate sweetened or sugary foods like candy, confectionery items, and ice cream while getting treated for Candida or a yeast infection. Also avoid flour-based eatables, such as bagels, bread, and pizza.

Also, make sure that you do not eat mushrooms, and avoid drinks including dairy, fermented drinks, alcoholic beers, champagne, and hard ciders involving apple cider vinegar. Get rid of fermented foods. For example, sauerkraut, kombucha, kimchi, kefir, and yogurt.

Now we are going to share some tried and tested food recipes to help you deal with yeast infections effectively. The first recipe we are going to share with you consists of bone broth that you can easily make in an instant pot. Here are the ingredients you need to prepare a juicy bone broth:

Instant Pot Bone Broth

INGREDIENTS

- 4 pounds beef bones
- A half an onion, cut
- A head of garlic, unpeeled
- 1 bay leaf
- 1 tablespoon apple cider vinegar
- At least one teaspoon Celtic sea salt, to taste

INSTRUCTIONS

1. Take a baking sheet and put the beef bones on it.
2. Roast them for 60 minutes at 350 F.
3. Transfer the bones from the oven to the instant pot.
4. Put the bay leaf, garlic, onion, vinegar, and the salt in the instant pot.
5. Fill water in the pot below max-fill line.
6. Put on the lid and lock it.
7. Set the high pressure manually, for 90 minutes.
8. Remove the lid and let it cool down.

Once the bone broth has been prepared, you can refrigerate it in one quart mason jars for 4 days, as well as freeze for up to 6 months.

If you are looking to eat salad, you have the option to make asparagus salad with basil leaves and tomatoes. It is incredibly delicious and the best item during the summers, especially if you are dealing with candida. Here are the ingredients to help you make 4 servings:

Asparagus Salad with Basil Leaves

INGREDIENTS

- 1 pound of asparagus, cut into 1 inch pieces (shed the fibrous end)
- 1 cup grape tomatoes, halved
- 1 ripe avocado, cut into cubes
- 1 cup basil leaves, sliced
- 1/4 cup olive oil
- 2 teaspoons lemon juice
- 2 teaspoons Dijon mustard
- ½ teaspoon Celtic Sea salt
- ½ teaspoon of ground black pepper

INSTRUCTIONS

1. Steam the asparagus for five to seven minutes.
2. Take a large bowl and place basil, avocado, tomatoes, and asparagus in it.
3. Take the olive oil and stir the mustard and lemon juice in it.
4. Sprinkle some pepper and salt.

It is ready to eat. You can create portions and share them with four people.

Further, you may have heard about green eggs and how effective they could be when it comes to dealing with a yeast infection. Let's help you add more power to your nutrition by sharing the secret recipe for cooking green eggs. Here are the ingredients you need:

Green Eggs

INGREDIENTS FOR TWO SERVINGS

- 4 Large eggs
- 4 Large kale leaves, do not remove the stems
- a pinch of Celtic sea salt
- Oil—depends on your choice and the frying pan you use

INSTRUCTIONS

1. Place the kale, salt, and eggs in a blender.
2. Blend the ingredients on high until smooth.
3. In an 8-inch frying pan heat the oil on medium heat.
4. Pour the egg mixture in the pan.
5. Cook the eggs as per your requirement.
6. Enjoy the dish.

Being religiously on a Candida diet could be quite monotonous as far as your eating options are concerned. As you eat the same food interchangeably, a time may come when you start hating the leafy greens and crave fast and processed food. At the same time, you need to realize that nothing is worth more than your health. Being on a strict diet for a few weeks could frustrate you, but in the long run, that is the only choice you have if you are serious about healing from Candida.

It is an infection and may trouble you for a while, causing your skin to itch and develop rashes, but the good thing is it is curable as well as preventable. It may also teach you something valuable about your body and help you cooperate with it. You will learn to give healthier nutrition to your body, and it is a universal fact that as you sow, so shall you reap.

The same is true with your body. If you keep feeding it with all sorts of toxic substances, it is naturally going to protest in the form of developing an illness. In other words, when you have an illness, it is a way for your body to tell you how you are abusing it. Once you genuinely listen to what your body is communicating with you, you will take precautionary measures to heal it and never repeat the mistake.

Therefore, when you feed your body with healthy foods and lots of water, it rewards you with radiating and glowing skin, making you appear physically, spiritually, and mentally healthy. It is true that the kind of food you eat has a lot to do with the way your body appears. You feed it with crap, and it gives the crap back to you and vice versa. Remember to treat your body well so that it treats you in the same way.

CHAPTER 7

Nutritional Recipes to Support Autism and Other Disorders

Autism is a brain disorder that makes it hard for an individual to communicate and interact with others. A child is brought into the world with autism or the inclination to foster it. At this moment, it's not something you can forestall, unfortunately. Autism is the most widely recognized of a gathering of related disorders called autistic spectrum disorders (ASDs). The most common autistic spectrum disorder is Asperger's syndrome, which is also momentarily portrayed in this handout. While ASD is now and again diagnosed in an adult, these disorders are most frequently recognized and diagnosed in childhood.

Individuals with autism have at least one symptom in each area listed below. While many of these symptoms appear in youth, autism warning signs can be found in babies.

How is Autism Diagnosed?

There's no single test to diagnose autism. Instead, doctors depend on the accompanying:

- *Checklists and questionnaires:* from parents, school professionals, and medical specialists who have observed the individual in various situations. The questionnaires ask about the individual's behaviors, relationships with others, body use, verbal communication, and play habits.

- *Standard medical criteria*: A doctor diagnoses autism provided that the information gathered fulfills guideline criteria for the disorder. Using the checklists and questionnaires above, your doctor gathers this information by talking to and observing your youngster.

- *Medical tests*: Additional tests may be utilized to get more information. These tests don't "diagnose" autism; in any case, they can take care of rules or discover different circumstances that may be causing symptoms (or making them worse).

- *Hearing evaluations:* To rule out hearing problems, and discourse and language evaluations to assess discourse, language, and overall communication abilities. These evaluations are vital because autism significantly impacts overall communication abilities.

- *Evaluation by specialists*: Talking with at least one specialist can frequently be useful in the complicated course of diagnosing autism.

What Causes Autism?

Autism was first distinguished in 1943. However, we don't have the foggiest idea what causes it. Since individuals are brought into the world with autism or have the potential to foster it, scientists are concentrating on hereditary and environmental factors.

- *Hereditary factors*: Scans show contrasts in brain shape and construction in individuals with autism. Scientists think these changes are hereditary.

- *Environmental factors*: On the off chance that an individual has a hereditary inclination toward autism, certain environmental factors may "trigger" it. Factors considered include viral contaminations, metabolic imbalances, and openness to certain chemicals.

- *NOT vaccines*: There are NO demonstrated connections between vaccines and autism. Research studies have repeatedly shown identical autism rates for patients who have gotten vaccines (like the polio vaccine or MMR) or vaccine preservatives (like thimerosal) and patients who have not gotten them.

How are autism spectrum disorders treated? Studies show that early, individualized, and escalated treatment has the best impact on the abilities of an individual with autism. Therapy for explicit functional problems could start before a formal diagnosis is received. Since no single strategy works with each individual, individualized treatment strategies are used to meet an individual's special needs. A concentrated approach means a patient engages actively and gainfully in meaningful activities for at least 25 hours of the week—with a treatment provider, family, caregivers, or teachers. Each strategy below aims at the same overall goal: diminishing symptoms and assisting the individual with autism to prevail in various settings and relationships.

Behavioral and Communication Training

A variety of approaches can assist individuals with ASDs change behavior and further develop communication abilities:

- *SCERTS Model*: This model addresses key areas of weakness for ASDs, like social communication (SC) and emotional regulation (ER), along with assisting caregivers with giving transaction supports (TS) that expand on a child's assets. The SCERTS model assists families with incorporating abilities learned in treatment into the family's everyday routines (for example, getting dressed, meals, or playtime).

- *Applied Behavioral Analysis (ABA) or Early and Intensive Behavioral Intervention (EIBI):* Traditional ABA utilizes profoundly organized teaching activities that focus on clear educational ideas. Contemporary ABA is more adaptable; it utilizes positive behavioral support and incidental teaching (teaching that happens inside continuous activities and is based on the understudy's advantage and motivation). Treatment includes as long as 40 hours a day seven days a week, for two years.

- *Project TEACCH (Treatment and Education of Autistic and Related Communication-Handicapped Children)*: This classroom-based model spotlights accommodating the learning styles of children with ASDs. It downplays distractions, utilizes pictures and visual prompts to reinforce learning, and uses an exceptionally organized plan.

- *Parent-driven treatment*: RDI (Relationship Development Intervention) and DIR (Developmental, Individual-Difference, Relationship-Based Model). These programs are based on a parent coaching model—a consultant teaches parents and family individuals who work with the child. Play-focused therapy emphasizes the child's advantages and interactions between child and parent. "Floor time" exercises aim to assist children with further developing abilities in attention, communication, and logical idea.

- *Sensory Integration Therapy*: This occupational therapy model assists individuals with autism in integrating and involving sensory information into daily life. Occupational therapy with this approach assists individuals with working on emotional regulation and motor abilities for daily living and play.

- *The Listening Program*: When joined with different approaches, this music-based program can assist individuals with working on their abilities in handling sounds.

- *PECS (Picture Exchange Communication System) and other visual strategies*: For children who battle communicating with language, these strategies assist them with communicating by exchanging pictures.

- *Video modeling*: With this teaching technique, target behaviors are videotaped, and the child watches the videotapes to memorize and imitate the behaviors.

Treatment of Different Problems

Many children with autism face other developmental problems. The most well-known are attention shortage/hyperactivity disorder (ADHD), anxiety, learning disabilities, despair, and bipolar disorder. These can lead to symptoms that are often treated with medication:

- *Medication to reduce tantrums, self-injury, or aggression*: Your doctor may recommend risperidone (Risperdal) or a similar medication if your child has an issue with serious tantrums or aggression.

- *Medication to reduce hyperactivity or lack of attention*: Children with autism sometimes have problems zeroing in on tasks and want to be moving all the time. Your doctor may recommend medication to assist your child with centering.

- *Medication to reduce anxiety, tedious behaviors, or routines:* To address these symptoms, your doctor may recommend appropriate medication. Several alternatives exist, so if the principal medication recommended doesn't help, your doctor could endorse an alternate one. Individuals with autism often face other explicit medical problems, and treating them can reduce ASD symptoms. Talk to your care team if you notice any of these:

- *Hardships with eating:* Children with ASDs can take "demanding eating" to the limit—denying food varieties based on texture or type or eating unambiguous food sources.

- *Gastrointestinal problems:* Individuals with ASDs can have cramps, diarrhea, and bloating.

- *Rest disturbances:* Individuals with ASDs often have difficulty falling asleep or waking early in the morning. After attempting therapy or medication, if your child keeps battling with the problems listed above —assuming they disrupt relationships or routines at home, school, work, or with companions—talk with your doctor about consulting a mental health provider who specializes in autism spectrum disorders.

Alternative Approaches

'What else can we do? We'll take a stab at anything.' As a parent, you may feel as such, and you'll probably hear or read about many therapies in addition to those portrayed in this booklet. These are often considered "alternative therapies" and incorporate vitamin therapy, special eating regimens, and others. Be careful with alternative therapies. Most alternative therapies have NOT been tried in logical examinations. A few therapies are dangerous, like chelation (using chemicals to eliminate metals from the body). Different therapies are costly and ineffectual, like treatment with the hormone secretin. A presence of mind approach? Try not to act like a lone ranger. For your child's sake, discuss any alternative therapy you are thinking about with your child's treatment team. For different tips, see the panel at the right.

An optimal eating regimen is balanced and loaded with supplements. This can sometimes be challenging for autistic individuals since many have stomach-related issues. Individuals with autism are often deficient in certain supplements, so a food list for autism will incorporate food sources like plant oil products, nuts, beans, eggs, and lean meats.

A few food varieties may cause gastrointestinal issues in autistic children. At times, carrying out a specialized eating routine, for example, a gluten-free/without casein or ketogenic diet, may work well. Working with your pediatrician and potentially a nutritionist is important to expand your child's eating routine.

Eating Optimal Foods: Autistic Children and Problems with Food

Children with autism often have scanty sustenance, partly because of food avoidance and aversions. Poor nutrition increases the risk of later ailments, like diabetes and heart disease. Children who grow up with poor eating regimens are more prone to being large, which is associated with several constant ailments.

Children with autism are more prone to low calcium and protein, which reduces brain advancement, bone development, and muscle strength. These issues may be correlated with problems with cognizance, balance, physical strength, and different aspects of physical change.

Taking care of issues can be a major problem for autistic children, and the results can be serious if the child winds up with nutritional lacks. Parents can help by utilizing various strategies to get their children to eat a different regimen. Doctors and therapists are often engaged in this interaction.

Autism and Dietary Struggles

Why is autism often attached to dietary battles?

Individuals on the autism spectrum have a developmental condition that manifests in various behavioral contrasts and challenges. These can sometimes become obvious when taking care of problems. An autistic individual's issues with food may manifest as:

- Rituals around eating
- Taking food in their cheeks or sucking on food instead of biting it
- Firmly inclining toward certain food varieties
- Avoiding certain food varieties

Individuals with autism are also at higher risk for gastrointestinal problems. Autistic children may also avoid certain food sources or foster solid texture or temperature aversions because of sensory issues.

In frustration, parents of autistic children may restrict their child's food sources to those they realize will be accepted. Be that as it may, this is not a sustainable model for fostering healthy eating and nourishment habits.

As you work with your child's pediatrician and a nutritionist, you can start to expand your child's eating regimen. After some time, you and your child's treatment team can foster a list of optimal food sources that your child appreciates and a list of food sources to avoid that often bring about stomach-related issues.

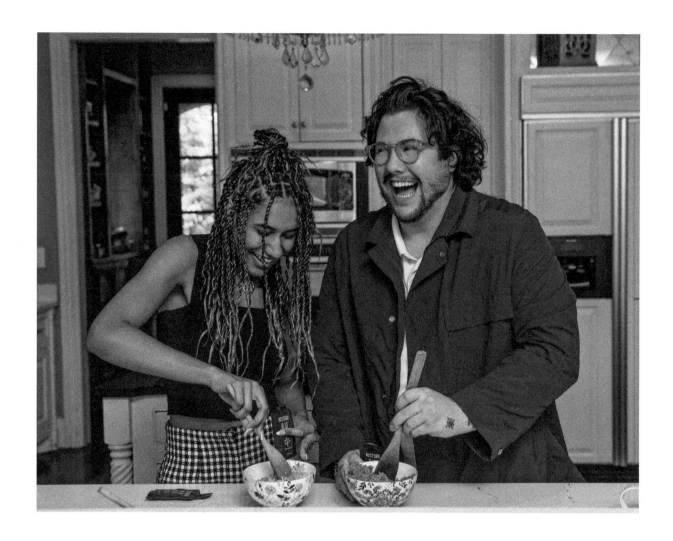

Diets to Support Positive Behaviors and Healthy Eating

Many parents with autistic children go to specialists to support their child's health. Several examinations have shown that children with autism will generally avoid healthier food sources, similar to vegetables and new natural products, in favor of more processed starches and snack food sources. They may also battle to get sufficient protein, as the texture of several food sources containing protein may be unappealing.

To encourage change in these behaviors, parents often attempt certain approaches to taking care of problems. These are the three most normal eating regimens for autism:

Autism MEAL Plan: This is not only a nutritional plan, as parents can train in this behavioral approach so they can offer the best assistance to their children. Behavior therapies are often among the best approach to addressing and taking care of problems in individuals with autism. The autism MEAL plan centers on changing behaviors toward certain food varieties.

This is, as yet, a relatively new approach to assisting children with autism to get their nutritional requirements met. A few examinations offered parents training in autism MEAL plans for about two months and found that the behavioral approach eased caregiver stress around mealtimes a great deal. Nonetheless, it was noticed that children with autism didn't have behavioral upgrades around meals or food selectivity.

Further research is yet to be expected to understand in the event that applying this particular behavioral approach can assist children with long naming or assuming there is a restricted advantage to the approach.

Sans gluten/without casein diet (GFCF): Many parents put their children on the GFCF diet, especially parents of autistic children. Since both gluten, a wheat protein, and casein, a dairy protein, can make stomach-related problems in autistic individuals worse, eliminating these from a child's eating routine can appear to make sense, yet there is deficient research to support this idea.

The gluten/sans casein diet may further develop behaviors around nourishment for some time, yet it tends to be challenging to make sure your child gets sufficient protein, entire grains, and amino acids, which are often part of bread and dairy in Western eating regimens. It's important to find other food choices to address these issues.

Altered ketogenic diet: This low-carbohydrate, moderate-protein, high-fat eating routine can assist children with autism get the required protein for brain and muscle advancement while eliminating potential wellsprings of stomach-related discomfort, like wheat. An emphasis on certain sorts of protein can try and assist you with eliminating dairy from your child's eating routine in the event that cheddar cheese or milk causes them stomach-related distress.

Since this diet is attached to higher supplement intake while eliminating certain irritants, it very well may be more viable for autistic children than different weight control plans. It is important to be careful of the amount of fat that is eaten, as this can add to heart disease and weight, especially assuming your child battles to eat other healthy food sources, like products of the soil.

Is There an Optimal Food List for Autistic Children?

An investigation discovered that the most well-known supplement deficiencies in children with autism were fiber, folic acid, calcium, iron, zinc, and vitamins A, C, D, E, K, B6, and B12.

Because of food inclinations or fixations, a few children may need a lot of or a couple of these supplements. Food avoidances mean that many autistic children need more of these vitamins and minerals.

To assist your child with getting the right balance of these important supplements, try adding these food sources to their eating regimen with the assistance of their treatment team:

- Beans—like navy beans, pinto beans, and black beans
- Peanuts and peanut butter
- Sunflower seeds
- Eggs
- Seafood
- Chia seeds
- Soy milk
- Almonds and almond milk
- Dried figs and apricots
- Edamame
- Cruciferous vegetables, like kale and broccoli
- Spinach
- Fortified breakfast cereal
- Lentils
- Dark chocolate, as an occasional sweet treat
- Lean meat, turkey, and chicken
- Chickpeas
- Oatmeal
- Green peas
- Mango
- Melons, like cantaloupe
- Tomatoes and tomato juice
- Carrots
- Sweet red pepper
- Pumpkin
- Citrus, like oranges and grapefruit
- Mushrooms
- Beet greens
- Butternut squash

- Avocado
- Rice
- Onions and garlic

Many of these food sources offer various supplements, so joining them in various ways through meal planning can assist your child with getting excellent supplements, avoiding food varieties that cause discomfort, and gradually adding new encounters to your child's eating habits.

Start planning meals that contain several natural products, vegetables, grains, and proteins, so there is a variety of choices. Sprinkle in new food sources with reliable choices you realize your child will like.

Potential Foods to Avoid

In the event that you notice a particular food brings about stomach issues or negative behaviors, avoid it. These are normal food varieties that may cause issues in children with autism:

- Milk and other dairy items
- Wheat items
- High-sugar food sources
- Processed meats

Veggie Burger Recipe

INGREDIENTS

- 1 can pinto or black beans (other varieties also work)
- 3 tablespoons tomato paste or ketchup
- 1/2 teaspoon salt
- 1/2 teaspoon garlic powder, optional
- 1/4 teaspoon onion powder
- 2 tablespoons flour of choice or oat bran
- 1/2 cup cooked diced vegetables of choice

INSTRUCTIONS

1. These burgers can be baked, grilled, or fried, and feel free to use whatever veggies you have on hand. For the burgers in the pictures, use roasted mushrooms, asparagus, and onion. You can also change up the flavor by adding different spices, such as paprika, cumin, or curry powder.

2. To make the veggie burgers, first drain, rinse, and mash the beans either by hand or in a food processor, depending on desired burger texture.

3. Stir in all other ingredients, and form patties. (Add more flour if too soft to form patties.) Either pan fry–flipping halfway through cooking–or place on a parchment-lined pan and bake at 350 F for 10 minutes.

4. Flip, then bake an additional 10 minutes or until desired texture is reached. (You can also grill the burgers. Leftovers can be refrigerated or frozen in meal prep containers for a later day.

Stuffed Cucumber Salad

INGREDIENTS:

- 2 medium-sized cucumbers
- 1 big, boiled potato
- 1 tablespoon soaked yellow moong dal, coarsely grinded
- 1 tablespoon coriander leaves
- Salt to taste
- ¼ teaspoon fresh lemon juice
- 1 teaspoon oregano

METHOD:

1. Cut cucumber vertically.
2. Scoop out seeds.
3. Mix all other ingredients in a bowl. You can use the seeds of cucumber also (optional)
4. Stuff the mixture in the cucumber.
5. Chill and serve.

BISCUITS

INGREIDENTS:

- ½ cup brown rice flour, 65 grams
- ½ cup sorghum flour, 65 grams
- 1 tablespoon flax seed meal (optional)
- 2 teaspoons baking powder
- 1/3 cup vegetable shortening or plant-based butter
- 1 teaspoon baking soda
- ½ teaspoon salt

INSTRUCTIONS:

1. Preheat oven to 375 °F. Lightly grease a baking sheet.
2. In a medium-sized bowl, combine all dry ingredients. Stir.
3. Add shortening and mix until mixture resembles a fine crumb.
4. Mix well until combined into a pasty, soft dough. It will be quite fragile. Pat out dough on the baking sheet to 1/2-inch thickness.
5. Cut into square biscuits and push apart with the side of the knife. Bake for 15 to 20 minutes, depending upon thickness, until the biscuits have browned and are cooked through.

Bread Loaf

INGREDIENTS:

- ⅔ cup brown rice flour, 80 grams
- ⅓ cup sorghum flour, 45 grams
- ⅓ cup canola oil
- 1 tablespoon flaxseed meal
- 2 tablespoons honey
- 1 teaspoon apple cider vinegar
- 2 eggs (omega-3 enriched)
- 1 tablespoon baking powder
- ½ teaspoon baking soda
- 1 teaspoon xanthan gum
- ½ teaspoon salt
- ½ cup apple juice

INSTRUCTIONS:

1. Preheat oven to 350 °F. Lightly grease a medium-sized loaf pan.
2. In a mixing bowl, combine flours and oil. Mix well to combine. Add remaining ingredients and mix well. Batter will thicken as it is beaten. Pour into loaf pan.
3. Smooth top with moistened fingertips for a prettier loaf, if desired.
4. Bake for approximately 30 minutes, until a toothpick inserted in the middle tests clean.

Easy Dinner Rolls

INGREDIENTS:

- ⅔ cup brown rice flour, 80 grams
- ⅓ cup sorghum flour, 45 grams
- ⅓ cup canola oil 2 tablespoons
- 1 teaspoon honey
- 1 tablespoon of apple cider vinegar
- 2 eggs (omega-3 enriched)
- 1 tablespoon baking powder
- ½ teaspoon baking soda
- ¾ teaspoon xanthan gum
- ½ teaspoon cinnamon
- ½ teaspoon salt
- 1 teaspoon ground flaxseed meal

INSTRUCTIONS:

1. Preheat oven to 350 °F.
2. Lightly grease a 12-cup muffin tin.
3. In a mixing bowl, combine flours and oil.
4. Mix well to combine.
5. Add the remaining ingredients and mix well. Batter will thicken as it is beaten. Divide batter among cups in the tin.
6. Bake for approximately 15 to 18 minutes, until a toothpick inserted in the middle tests clean.

Nutritional Recipes to Support Dementia, Alzheimer's Disease, Parkinson's Disease, and ALS

Dementia and Alzheimer's disease aren't similar. Dementia is a general term used to portray side effects that influence memory, the performance of daily activities, and correspondence capacities. Alzheimer's disease is the most widely recognized kind of dementia, and Alzheimer's disease deteriorates with time, and influences memory, language, and thought.

While more youthful individuals can foster dementia or Alzheimer's, your risk increases as you age. Dementia and Alzheimer's disease is most common in adults older than 65, and it is viewed as a standard piece of adulating.

Side effects of the two circumstances can overlap, yet recognizing them is significant for management and treatment. Continue to research to find out about the distinctions.

What is Dementia?

The World Health Organization (WHO) assesses that more than 55 million individuals worldwide are living with dementia.

Dementia is a disorder, not a disease. A disorder is a gathering of side effects that don't have a conclusive determination. Dementia influences mental undertakings, like memory and thinking, which can happen because of different circumstances. The most well-known of which is Alzheimer's disease.

Individuals can have more than one sort of dementia, and this is known as mixed dementia. Individuals with mixed dementia have side effects of at least two sorts of dementia. A finding of mixed dementia must be affirmed in an examination.

As dementia advances, it can colossally affect the capacity to work freely. It's a significant reason for the inability of older adults and puts a close-to-home and monetary weight on families and guardians. Dementia is additionally the fifth driving reason for death "WHO" around the world, and cases are supposed to increase significantly over the next 30 years.

The early side effects of dementia are not entirely obvious but can be gentle. Dementia often starts with straightforward episodes of forgetfulness. Individuals with dementia experience difficulty monitoring time and generally become lost in recognizable settings.

As dementia advances, forgetfulness and confusion develop. It becomes harder to review names and faces. Individual recognition turns into an issue. Clear indications of dementia incorporate repetitious questioning, lacking cleanliness, and issue with direction.

In the most advanced stage, individuals with dementia become unfit to focus on themselves. They will experience more difficulty monitoring time and recollecting individuals and places they know about. Their way of behaving can proceed to change and can transform into discouragement and animosity.

Reasons for Dementia

You're bound to foster dementia as you age. It happens when certain synapses are damaged. Many circumstances can cause dementia, including degenerative diseases like Alzheimer's, Parkinson's, and Huntington's. Each reason for dementia causes damage to an alternate arrangement of synapses. Alzheimer's disease is answerable for around 60 to 80 percent of all instances of dementia.

Different reasons for dementia include:

- contaminations, like HIV
- vascular diseases
- stroke
- sadness
- constant medication use

According to the Centers for Disease Control and Prevention (CDC), older African Americans are twice as likely to foster dementia as non-Hispanic white individuals. Hispanic individuals are 1.5 times more likely to have dementia than non-Hispanic white individuals. One justification for these measurements might be fundamental disparities and hindrances to medical services for minimized groups.

What is Alzheimer's Disease?

Dementia is the term applied to various side effects that adversely influence memory. Yet, Alzheimer's is a particular moderate disease of the mind that gradually causes disability in memory and mental capability. The specific reason is obscure, and no fix is accessible. Although, more youthful individuals can and do get Alzheimer's—the side effects, for the most part, start after age 65.

The Impacts of Alzheimer's on the Mind

In individuals with Alzheimer's disease, synapses bite the dust, and associations between synapses might differ. One of the trademark side effects is unusual protein stores in the brain, called plaques and tangles. Plaques are thick groups of protein that can hinder correspondence between neurons, and tangles are proteins that turn together, leading to the passing of solid synapses.

In cutting-edge Alzheimer's, the cerebrum shows critical shrinkage. Changes in the cerebrum might happen a decade or more before side effects start.

It's difficult to determine whether Alzheimer's has total exactness while an individual is alive. The conclusion must be affirmed when the brain is inspected under a magnifying lens during a post-mortem examination. In any case, experts can make the right finding up to 90 percent of the time.

The side effects of Alzheimer's and dementia can overlap. However, there can be a few distinctions.

The Two Circumstances Can Cause:
- a decrease in the capacity to think
- memory loss
- communication impairment

The Side Effects of Alzheimer's Include:
- trouble reflecting on ongoing occasions or discussions
- apathy
- melancholy
- hindered judgment
- bewilderment
- confusion
- behavioral changes
- trouble talking, gulping, or walking in cutting-edge stages of the disease

A few kinds of dementia will share a portion of these side effects. However, they incorporate or prohibit different side effects that can assist with making a differential conclusion.

For instance, Lewy body dementia (LBD) has many similar later side effects as Alzheimer's. Be that as it may, individuals with LBD are bound to encounter initial side effects like visual pipedreams, hardships with equilibrium, and unsettling sleep influences.

Individuals with dementia because of Parkinson's or Huntington's disease are bound to encounter compulsory development in the beginning phases of the disease.

How is Alzheimer's Versus Dementia Treated?

Treatment for dementia will rely upon the specific reason and kind of dementia; there are numerous medicines for dementia and Alzheimer's out there for patients to try, even though no solution for Alzheimers is accessible; however, choices to assist with overseeing side effects of the disease include:

- medications for behavioral changes, like antipsychotics
- medications for memory loss, which incorporate cholinesterase inhibitors donepezil (Aricept) and rivastigmine (Exelon), and memantine (Namenda)
- elective cures that mean to help brain capability or, generally, for well-being, like coconut oil or fish oil
- medications for sleep changes
- medications for despondency

Dementia Treatment

At times, treating the condition that causes dementia might help. Conditions likely to respond to treatment incorporate dementia brought about by:

- drugs
- cancers
- metabolic problems
- hypoglycemia

Generally speaking, dementia isn't reversible. Notwithstanding, many forms are treatable. The right prescription can assist with overseeing dementia. Medicines for dementia will rely upon the reason. For instance, specialists often treat dementia brought about by Parkinson's disease, Alzheimer's, and LBD with cholinesterase inhibitors.

Treatment for vascular dementia will zero in on preventing further damage to the brain's blood vessels and preventing stroke. Individuals with dementia can likewise profit from steady administration from home well-being helpers and guardians. A helping office or nursing home might be fundamental as the disease advances.

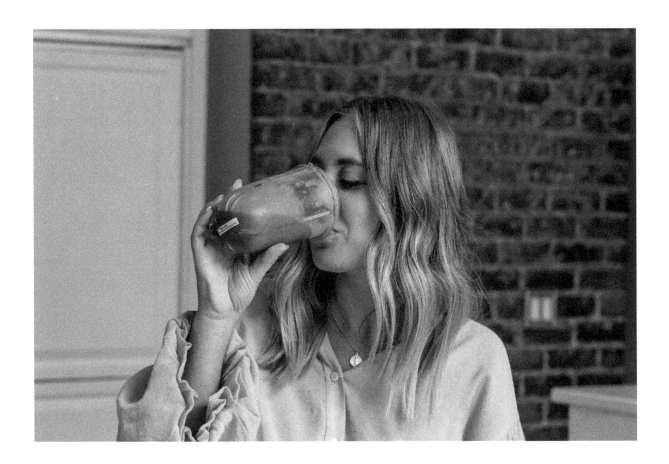

How Does the MIND Diet Work to Boost Brain Health?

The MIND diet centers around the admission of plant-based food sources and restricting the admission of animal products and food varieties high in saturated fat. The accentuation is on plants, and what's critical is that this diet explicitly encourages a higher utilization of berries and green leafy vegetables.

Energizing up with flavonoid-rich produce may for sure help the mind. Blueberries, strawberries, and blackberries seem to forestall mental maturing in women by up to two years, per an initial concentration distributed in the *Annals of Neurology*. In like manner, there's a connection between eating leafy green vegetables—like kale, spinach, and collard greens—and lower irritation and oxidative pressure, two factors that are related to Alzheimer's disease, per a past report distributed in the *Journal of the Academy of Nutrition and Dietetics*. These foods are wealthy in cell reinforcements and can assist with decreasing aggravation and oxidative pressure.

Oxidative pressure happens when cell reinforcement safeguards are low, and the body can't battle toxic molecules, called free radicals. This pressure causes cell damage in the brain and all through the body, and it has been connected with a few diseases, including Alzheimer's and malignant growth.

Dementia and Alzheimer's disease are believed to be brought about by a mix of hereditary, ecological, and way of life factors, including diet and nutrition. Ailments, for example, hypertension, heart disease, diabetes, and excess weight, may add to mental degradation and are often impacted by the food varieties you eat. Practicing great nutrition and eating heaps of good food varieties are displayed to assist with lessening your risk of dementia and Alzheimer's disease as you become older.

Not all reviews have shown a connection between eating great and a lift in discernment. In general, the proof recommends, however, doesn't demonstrate that following a Mediterranean or comparable diet could assist with lessening the risk for Alzheimer's dementia or slow mental degradation. To figure out more, researchers upheld by the National Institutes of Health (NIA) and different associations are directing clinical preliminaries—thought about the highest quality level of clinical proof—to reveal more insight into any circumstances and logical results.

While researchers don't as yet know why the Mediterranean diet could help the brain, its impact on developing cardiovascular well-being could lessen dementia risk. That's what two ongoing investigations propose. As a feature of this diet, eating fish might be the most grounded factor impacting higher mental capability and slower mental deterioration. Conversely, the standard Western diet increases cardiovascular disease risk, conceivably adding to quicker brain maturing.

Moreover, the Mediterranean diet could increase explicit supplements that might safeguard the brain through calming and cell-reinforcement properties. It might likewise repress beta-amyloid stores, which are found in the brains of individuals with Alzheimer's, or work on cell digestion in manners that safeguard against the disease.

For example, numerous food varieties—blueberries, leafy greens, and curcumin (found in turmeric)—have been studied for their expected mental advantage. These food sources were remembered to have mitigating, cell-reinforcement, or different properties that could assist with safeguarding the brain. Up to this point, there is no proof that eating or keeping away from a particular food can forestall Alzheimer's disease or age-related mental degradation.

In any case, researchers keep on searching for hints. One review, because older adults reported their dietary patterns, observed that eating a daily serving of leafy green vegetables, for example, spinach and kale, was related to slower age-related mental degradation, maybe because of the neuroprotective impacts of specific supplements. Research has likewise shown that a diet incorporating standard fish is related to higher mental capability and slower mental deterioration with age. One more late review, in mice, found that consuming a great deal of salt expanded levels of the protein tau, found in the brains of individuals with Alzheimer's, and caused mental weakness.

Here are food sources that can ward off mental degradation and assist you with remaining sound as you age:

Leafy Greens: Kale, collard greens, spinach, and Swiss chard are just a few of the leafy greens high in fundamental B nutrients like folate and B9 that can assist with diminishing discouragement while likewise helping perception. Rather than simply eating leafy greens in servings of mixed greens, add these stalwart vegetables to soups, stews, and you can likewise purèe them and add them to sauces, pesto, and hummus.

Berries: Raspberries, blueberries, blackberries, and cherries all contain a flavonoid called anthocyanin that stops the movement of brain damage set off by free radicals. These and different berries are likewise loaded with cell reinforcements and an abundance of nutrients that assist with diminishing irritation and assist you with keeping up with great brain well-being.

Nuts: Walnuts, almonds, pecans, cashews, and peanuts are loaded with solid fats, magnesium, vitamin E, and B nutrients—all displayed to advance great insight and avoid indications of dementia. Women over 70 years old should consume around 5 servings of nuts each week and are displayed to have fundamentally preferred brain well-being over women in a similar age group who don't eat nuts. Another review demonstrates how the calming phytochemicals in English pecans can lessen the irritation of brain cells to keep up with ideal brain well-being through the maturing system.

Omega-3s: Olive oil, flaxseeds, and greasy fish such as , salmon, and mackerel are instances of food varieties high in omega-3 unsaturated fats with DHA that assist your brain with remaining sound. Many examinations demonstrate that omega-3s are compelling at battling and preventing dementia and suggest taking 200 mg of DHA daily to accomplish great brain well-being. Notwithstanding, the average daily admission of DHA in the U.S. is assessed to be around 80 mg. Put forth a conscious attempt to consume higher measures of omega-3s or request that your primary care physician suggests protected, viable DHA supplements.

Cruciferous Vegetables: Broccoli, cauliflower, brussels sprouts, and other cruciferous vegetables are high in B nutrients and carotenoids that can lessen homocysteine levels—an amino acid connected to mental degradation, brain decay, and dementia. Try sautéeing cruciferous vegetables in garlic and olive oil, or sneak these superfoods into smoothies, soups, and sauces.

Spices: Spices like sage, cumin, and cinnamon taste incredible when used to prepare meals, and they additionally contain heaps of polyphenols—intensifies that offer various advantages for memory and brain well-being. Spices, for example, can destroy brain plaque and lessen aggravation to forestall mental debilitation and Alzheimer's. Begin filling your spice rack with various flavors that can perk up your dinners while keeping your brain solid.

Seeds: Sunflower, flax, and pumpkin seeds all contain cancer prevention agents and supplements like vitamin E, zinc, omega-3s, and choline that lessen mental deterioration. Nibble on the seeds themselves, sprinkle on servings of mixed greens, or slip them into treats like pudding and biscuits to profit from further developed brain well-being.

Beans: On the off chance that beans are not a customary piece of your diet, they ought to be. High in fiber and protein and low in calories and fat, they additionally assist with keeping your mind sharp as a component of the MIND diet. The specialists suggest eating beans three times each week to assist with lessening the risk of Alzheimer's.

Fish: The MIND diet concentrates on eating fish something like once every seven days safeguard brain capability. In any case, there's a compelling reason to overdo it; not at all like the Mediterranean diet, which suggests eating fish consistently; the MIND diet says once every seven days is sufficient.

Foods That Are Risk Factors for Alzheimer's

Many foods in the Western diet have been identified as risk factors for dementia and Alzheimer's, including red and processed meats, refined grains, sweets, and desserts. Excess alcohol intake, saturated fatty acids, and foods with a high number of calories are also risk factors for Alzheimer's. If you think that you or a loved one may be at risk for Alzheimer's, work with your doctor on developing a healthier diet and nutrition plan that greatly reduces the risk.

What About Vitamins and Supplements?

Observational studies and clinical trials have looked at many over-the-counter vitamins and dietary supplements, including vitamins B and E and ginkgo biloba, to prevent Alzheimer's disease or cognitive decline. The idea is that these dietary add-ons might attack oxidative damage or inflammation, protect nerve cells, or influence other biological processes involved in Alzheimer's.

Despite early findings of possible benefits for brain health, no vitamin or supplement has been proven to work in people. Overall, the evidence is weak as many studies were too small or too short to be conclusive.

Take DHA (docosahexaenoic acid), for example. Studies in mice showed that this omega-3 fatty acid, found in salmon and certain other fish, reduced beta-amyloid plaques, a hallmark of Alzheimer's. However, clinical trials in humans have had mixed results. In a study of 485 older adults with age-related cognitive decline, those who took a DHA supplement daily for 24 weeks showed improved learning and memory compared to those who took a placebo. Another study of 4,000 older adults—conducted primarily to study eye disease—concluded that taking omega-3 supplements, alone or with other supplements, did not slow cognitive decline.

At this time, no vitamin or supplement is recommended for preventing Alzheimer's or cognitive decline. Although widely available from drugstores and on the internet, many of these have not been tested for their effects on thinking. Their safety and effectiveness are largely unknown, and they may interact with other medications. (Note: A deficiency in vitamin B12 or folate may cause memory problems that are reversible with proper treatment.)

The idea of Alzheimer's as a metabolic disease that affects the brain, and Alzheimer's markers, such as glucose metabolism, have led scientists in various directions. Besides the Mediterranean diet and its variations, they are looking at other diets, as well as individual foods and nutrients.

For example, the ketogenic diet is a high-fat, low-carbohydrate diet that prompts the production of ketones, chemicals that help brain cells work. Studies show that this diet may affect gut bacteria in distinctive ways in people with and without cognitive impairment and may help brain cells better use energy, improving their overall function.

Socca Chickpea Pancakes

INGREDIENTS

- 2 cups chickpea flour (often sold with other products by Bob's Red Mill)
- 2 cups water (swap almond or nut milk for some of the water, for even more nutrients)
- 2 tablespoons extra virgin olive oil, plus more for the pan
- ¼ teaspoon kosher salt
- ¼ teaspoon black pepper, freshly ground
- ½ teaspoon turmeric, freshly grated or ground, optional

INSTRUCTIONS

1. Whisk all the ingredients together in a medium bowl. Set batter aside to rest for 10 minutes.
2. Warm 1 teaspoon olive oil in a a 6-inch nonstick skillet over medium heat. Pour in ⅓ cup socca batter and swirl to create an even pancake.
3. After about 2 minutes, air bubbles will appear on the surface of the socca. Use a spatula to release its edges from the pan, then carefully lift and turn over. (Be gentle! Socca are delicate and can easily tear, but they still taste delicious.) Cook on the other side for about 2 minutes, or until it is crispy and starting to brown.
4. Place finished socca on a plate. Eat as is, or topped with whatever you like. Pictured here: hummus, shredded cabbage, cilantro, and a sprinkling of Parmesan cheese.

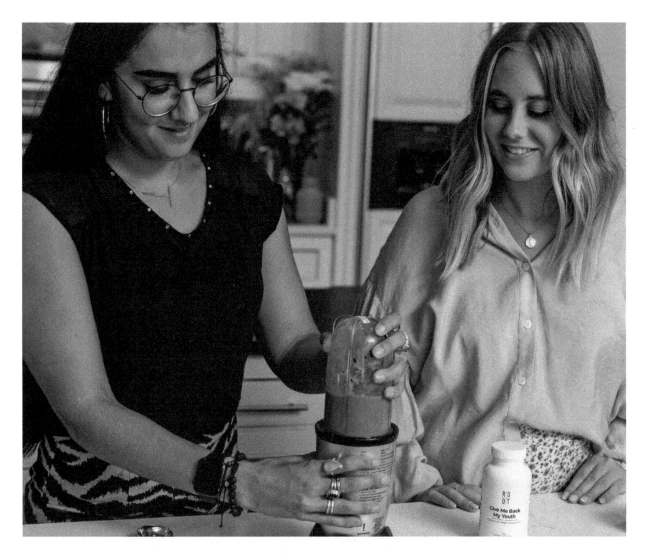

Brain Boosting Almond Butter and Blueberry Smoothie

INGREDIENTS

- 1 cup water
- 1 cup frozen wild blueberries
- 1 to 2 tablespoons unsweetened almond butter
- 2 scoops mamore, blueberry & lemon flavor
- 1 teaspoon Root Give Me Back My Youth (GMBMY)

INSTRUCTIONS

In a blender, add water, frozen blueberries, almond butter, and mamore. Purèe until well blended. If the smoothie is too thin in consistency, add ice until preferred consistency.

Panko Salmon & Spinach Salad

INGREDIENTS FOR PANKO-CRUSTED SALMON:

- Four 6 oz. salmon fillets
- 2 cups panko
- 1/2 cup parsley, finely chopped
- 1/2 teaspoon sea salt
- 1/2 teaspoon black pepper
- 2 tablespoons extra virgin olive oil
- 3 to 4 tablespoons Dijon mustard

INGREDIENTS FOR SPINACH SALAD:

- 2 handfuls mixed baby greens
- 2 handfuls spinach
- 8 to 10 cherry tomatoes
- 2 tablespoons balsamic vinegar
- 1 tablespoon honey
- 2 tablespoons olive oil
- 1/2 teaspoon Dijon mustard
- 1/4 teaspoon garlic powder

METHOD FOR PREPARING THE PANKO-CRUSTED SALMON:

1. Preheat the oven to 450°F (230°C).
2. Place a sheet of aluminum foil on a baking sheet, shiny side up.
3. In a medium bowl combine the panko, parsley, sea salt, fresh pepper, and extra virgin olive oil. With your hands, mix all the ingredients together, lightly crushing the panko into smaller pieces. Brush the top of the salmon fillets with a generous coat of Dijon mustard then coat it with the panko mixture, gently pushing it down to adhere to the mustard.
4. Arrange the fillets on the prepared baking sheet and bake them on the middle rack for 12 to 15 minutes. Rotate the baking sheet halfway through. While the salmon is in the oven, prepare the salad and salad dressing.

METHOD FOR PREPARING THE SPINACH SALAD:

1. Mix your baby greens and spinach together in a bowl. Slice the cherry tomatoes in half.

2. Combine balsamic vinegar, honey, extra virgin olive oil, Dijon mustard, and garlic in a bowl and mix well.

3. Drizzle over the salad. Place the salad on a plate with a slice or 2 of your salmon filet. Add a lemon wedge for the salmon, if you desire.

4. Enjoy!

Nutritional Recipes to Support Lyme Disease

Lyme disease is a bacterial infection that can be spread to humans by infected ticks. It's usually easier to treat when it's diagnosed early. Lyme disease is triggered by the bacterium Borrelia burgdorferi and, seldom, Borrelia mayonii. It is spread to humans through the bite of infected black-legged ticks. Typical symptoms include fever, headache, fatigue, and a characteristic skin rash called erythema migrans. Infection can spread to the joints, the heart, and the nervous system, if left untreated. Lyme disease is diagnosed based on symptoms, physical findings (e.g., rash), and possible exposure to infected ticks.

A circular- or oval-shaped rash around a tick bite can be an early side effect of Lyme disease in certain individuals. The rash can appear as long as 90 days after being bit by an infected tick; however, it usually appears within about a month and can last for a long time. The rash can have a darker or lighter area in the center and could gradually spread. It's not usually hot or itchy.

The rash may be flat or marginally raised and look pink, red, or purple when it appears on white skin. It may be harder to see the rash on brown and black skin, and it may seem like a bruise. There's no specific "Lyme disease diet" at this time. Fortunately, many people completely recover from Lyme disease after taking antibiotics.

Preliminary research recommends that certain plant oils have antibacterial effects that may support Lyme disease treatment and reduce waiting side effects. Additionally, anti-inflammatory compounds in certain foods may support your immune system to assist you with recovering from Lyme and different infections.

The Most Effective Method to Manage Inflammation in Lyme Disease

Infection with Borrelia burgdorferi, the bacterial cause of Lyme disease, and co-infections cause the immune system to launch a significant inflammatory reaction. While antibiotic treatments, such as doxycycline and cefuroxime, can annihilate B. burgdorferi, these medications do essentially nothing to mitigate the inflammatory reaction launched in light of these microbes. Left untreated, Lyme-induced inflammation damages cells, tissues, and organs, inducing widespread substantial dysfunction.

While the CDC gives recommendations for Lyme disease treatment according to the antimicrobial perspective, it makes no recommendations as to what is meant for individuals to manage the inflammatory symptoms of the sickness. Functional medicine, then again, offers a one-of-a-kind arrangement of instruments for managing Lyme-associated inflammation, including nourishment changes, way of life changes, and natural anti-inflammatory compounds. These holistic intercessions can significantly further develop Lyme disease inflammation, creating serious areas of strength for healing.

Swap the SAD Diet for an Anti-Inflammatory Diet

With regard to managing inflammation, a specific diet is a perfect place to start. The foods you choose to eat can either help or frustrate your recovery from Lyme disease by impacting your body's inflammatory weight. The Standard American Diet, rich in refined carbohydrates and industrial seed oils, increases the declaration of support of inflammatory cytokines, immune molecules that trigger an inflammatory reaction. Many of the same supportive inflammatory cytokines triggered by the SAD diet are also triggered by Lyme disease and other tick-borne infections. The SAD diet is also associated with an impaired immune reaction, which is the last thing you want while you're battling an infection. Other food groups, such as gluten and dairy, can also set off inflammation and are best avoided by individuals with Lyme disease.

Conversely, eating an anti-inflammatory, supplement-rich diet can accelerate your recovery and create a foundation for long-term health. At CCFM, we recommend that most patients start a Paleo reset diet. This diet is intended to reduce inflammation and develop assimilation, energy, glucose control, and body weight. The Paleo reset diet is centered on the following foods:

- Non-starchy vegetables—ideally 6 to 8 cups of vegetables across the color spectrum ("eat the rainbow")
- Whole organic products
- Pastured and organic meat, poultry, and eggs
- Seafood
- Starchy tubers, such as yams and cassava
- Organ meats, such as beef or chicken liver
- Bone stock
- Healthy fats such as extra virgin olive oil, coconut oil, coconut milk, avocado, nuts, and seeds

The Paleo reset diet is a strong strategy for reducing Lyme-related inflammation that can be additionally customized throughout your healing process, as required for your particular case. A portion of the additional nourishment intercessions that we most of the time prescribe on a case-by-case basis include:

- Autoimmune paleo diet (AIP)
- Low FODMAP diet
- Microbial reset diet
- Ketogenic diet
- Low histamine diet
- Low oxalate diet
- GAPS diet (a strong reset program in cases of extreme stomach inflammation)
- A gluten-free diet (gluten, dairy, soy, and corn are common trigger foods, among others)
- Elimination and reintroduction of diet
- Incorporate anti-inflammatory foods

To target Lyme-induced inflammation, you may also want to consider incorporating the following anti-inflammatory foods into your diet:

Omega-3 fatty acids: Preclinical research indicates that the omega-3 fatty acids EPA and DHA can balance the inflammatory reaction in Lyme disease by impacting populations of immune-signaling molecules. We recommend that Lyme patients consume at least 3 to 4 servings of fatty cold-water fish, preferably wild-caught, each week as a source of omega-3 fatty acids. While selecting seafood, utilize the acronym SMASH to recollect which kinds of seafood are the most supplement rich and lowest in mercury—salmon, mackerel, anchovies, sardines, and herring.

Cruciferous vegetables: Cruciferous vegetables such as broccoli and cauliflower give sulforaphane, a phytochemical that reduces inflammation via the anti-inflammatory Nrf2 cellular-signaling pathway. Activating the Nrf2 pathway creates glutathione, which your body needs to manage Lyme-induced inflammation and mount a healthy immune reaction. Microgreen and broccoli sprouts are also excellent sources of sulforaphane and are easy and enjoyable to make at home.

Matured foods: Fermented foods such as sauerkraut and kimchi contain probiotic bacteria and other bioactive compounds that reduce stomach inflammation and work on the immune system of the stomach, which has significant effects on systemic immune function.

Many individuals with tick-borne diseases battle with food-responsive qualities and gastrointestinal issues. Suppose you would like one-on-one assistance with your nourishment.

In that case, our staff nutritionist, Lindsay Christensen, can work with you to create a customized sustenance program to facilitate your healing process.

Sleep

Sleep disruption is a common side effect of Lyme disease. Be that as it may, excellent sleep is also essential for recovery because of its impacts on all body systems, especially the immune system and inflammation. A lack of sleep and poor-quality sleep taxes the immune system, while increasing inflammation. Improving your sleep is an essential move toward managing Lyme-associated inflammation.

Engaging in normal "sleep-hygiene" practices before bed can improve your sleep's therapeutic quality and may aid in reducing inflammation. Consider incorporating the following practices into your daily routine:

- Aim for 8-9 hours of sleep each evening. Research recommends that this is an ideal sleep target for most adults.

- Eat your last meal of the day at least three hours before bed. Eating excessively close to sleep time can reduce the therapeutic quality of your sleep.

- Wear blue-light-blocking glasses for at least an hour before bed. These glasses block out wavelengths of light that disrupt the production of the hormone melatonin. Your body needs melatonin to initiate and sustain sleep. Melatonin also has strong anti-inflammatory properties.

- Sleep in a dark, cool room. The ideal ambient temperature for sleep appears to be ~67 degrees Fahrenheit or colder.

- Create a relaxing sleep-time routine. Try doing a daily directed meditation or listening to soothing music before bed to assist your body with entering parasympathetic "rest, condensation, and repair" mode.

Anti-Inflammatory Interventions for Lyme

Past diet and sleep, several botanicals and nutraceuticals can be valuable for alleviating inflammation associated with Lyme and other tick-borne diseases.

Japanese Knotweed: This is a central component of several popular herbal protocols for Lyme disease. It is rich in resveratrol, a phytochemical with powerful anti-inflammatory properties.

Curcumin: This compound is found in dazzling orange turmeric root, a staple of traditional Chinese and Indian Ayurvedic medicine. Curcumin is a "prodigy" of the enhancement industry. For a valid justification, it has strong anti-inflammatory effects that make it an excellent alternative to NSAIDs for inflammation management and pain help.

Curcumin demonstrates significant advantages in alleviating arthritic inflammation and stomach and brain inflammation. Curcumin applies anti-inflammatory effects by blocking the activation of NF- B, a supportive inflammatory signaling pathway heavily involved in Lyme-induced inflammation.

Cat's Claw: Cat's Claw (Uncaria tomentosa) is a tropical climbing vine with sharp, curved thorns native to the Amazon rainforest of South America. The medicinal utilization of the inner bark of the vine dates back 2,000 years to the Inca civilization. Even today, Peruvian Ashaninka ministers regard the plant as sacred, using it for healing and in strict ceremonies.

Cat's Claw contains powerful alkaloid compounds with anti-inflammatory and antibacterial properties. Clinical trials indicate that the alkaloids found in Cat's Claw are particularly beneficial for alleviating inflammation by modulating the body's immune reaction. These findings recommend that Cat's Claw alkaloids may also mitigate arthritic side effects in chronic inflammatory conditions, such as Lyme disease.

CBD: Cannabidiol (CBD), a non-psychoactive phytocannabinoid in the hemp plant, also offers strong anti-inflammatory properties. It can further inhibit inflammation in the musculoskeletal, brain, and gastrointestinal tract, targeting different body systems impacted by Lyme and other tick-borne diseases.

Glutathione: This functions as a vital antioxidant throughout the body, including within the sensory system, and it also plays important jobs in detoxification. The immune system requires glutathione to mount an attack against Borrelia burgdorferi; subsequently, glutathione levels in chronic Lyme patients can become exhausted over the long haul. Supplemental glutathione and supplements like alpha lipoic acid (ALA) and N-acetyl cysteine (NAC) can help support glutathione and reduce inflammation caused by Lyme, as well as support the immune system. Eating a diet with plenty of sulfur-rich foods such as cruciferous vegetables, vitamin C, and selenium can also assist with boosting your body's natural glutathione production.

Anti-Inflammatory Strategies Work in Synergy with Antimicrobial Treatments

Inflammation management is essential to a comprehensive Lyme and TBD treatment protocol. Treating the infection without managing the inflammatory reaction can make antimicrobial treatment challenging to tolerate; conversely, implementing strategies that alleviate inflammation can make your Lyme treatment experience much more effective and comfortable. Our clinicians at CCFM are experienced in helping patients navigate

Lyme-induced inflammation during the treatment process and can assist you with selecting the best comprehensive anti-inflammatory interventions to address your issues.

There is no standard diet recommendation for treating Lyme disease. However, you could eat foods that would probably work on physical side effects and your overall health. Eating a diet that would minimize oxidation and inflammation could be of advantage.

We cannot stop oxidation, as it occurs from breathing in oxygen. However, you can certainly minimize it with diet. Excess oxidation increases the risk of all chronic diseases and aging and increases inflammation. Foods that would increase oxidation and inflammation:

Attempt to Avoid

Vegetable seed oils and foods made with them: Soybeans, safflower, corn oil, margarine, salad dressing, and mayonnaise. These foods are high in polyunsaturated fats, which easily oxidize. Canola oil wouldn't increase oxidation. However, it would also not further develop inflammation.

Red meat or hamburger: This would be all cuts of hamburger, including all ground hamburger (hamburger, cheeseburger, meatloaf, meatballs, American chop suey, meat chili, etc.). A polyunsaturated fat found in red meat (arachidonic acid) would increase oxidation.

Being overweight increases the inflammation in your body, and losing weight with a healthy diet and keeping it off will assist with decreasing inflammation.

Foods That Will Decrease Oxidation and Inflammation: (use foods rich in phenol oleocanthal and salicylic acid)

Extra Virgin Olive Oil (EVOO): This is the juice of the olive and has been related to improving many risk factors for chronic diseases. By definition, all EVOO is first squeezed, and cold squeezed. EVOO is mainly monounsaturated fat, so it doesn't easily oxidize, and it naturally has various antioxidants, and daily use has been displayed to decrease oxidation. The health advantages of EVOO are from the phenols that are found in all EVOO.

A few kinds of olive oil are rich in the phenol oleocanthal, which is a natural anti-inflammatory agent. Olive oil made from the Koroneki, Mission, Coratina, or Picholine olives is higher in oleocanthal content than other olives. The health advantages of EVOO start at 2 tablespoons a day. The most effective way to utilize EVOO is with vegetables; a decent guideline is 1 tablespoon of EVOO per cup of vegetables. Some foods grown from the ground are high in salicylic acid, a component found in aspirin, which can assist with decreasing inflammation. The following is a list of these foods:

Natural products: Apricots, berries (blackberry, blueberry, boysenberry, cranberry, loganberry, raspberry, strawberry), cantaloupe, cherries, grapes (and raisins), oranges, pineapple, and plum (and prunes).

Vegetables: Broccoli, cucumber, green peppers, okra, radishes, spinach, yams, processed tomatoes (all tomato products including ketchup and tomato sauce), and zucchini. A serving is ½ a cup of vegetables or natural product (which is very small, on the off chance that you like vegetables and not to an extreme, on the off chance that you don't); ¼ cup tomato sauce; 1 cup of salad greens; or ½ a cup or ½ a piece of organic product (so a piece of organic product is 2 servings). The goal would be nine servings of foods grown from the ground each day. This can easily be accomplished if you have a piece of organic product at breakfast and lunch, a 2-cup salad with lunch, and 1 ½ cup of vegetables at dinner. Remember that tomato sauce counts as a vegetable and is high in salicylic acid.

Carrot Almond Pancakes

- 1 cup peeled and grated carrots (2 to 3 carrots)
- ¼ cup almonds
- 1 slice fresh ginger (1/8-inch thick)
- 1 teaspoon ground flaxseed
- 2 tablespoons unsweetened shredded coconut
- ½ teaspoon ground cinnamon
- 1 egg
- ¼ teaspoon sea salt
- ½ teaspoon vanilla
- 1 to 2 tablespoons ghee (page 234)
- 1 teaspoon raw honey
- blueberries (optional)
- 1 teaspoon Root Give Me Back My Youth (GMBMY)

INSTRUCTIONS

1. Place the grated carrots in a medium-sized bowl.
2. Place the almonds, ginger, and flaxseed in the bowl of a food processor. Pulse 5 to 6 times until the almonds are finely ground.
3. Add the almond mixture and all of the remaining ingredients, except for the ghee, honey, and blueberries (if using), to the grated carrots.
4. Heat the ghee in a small frying pan over medium heat for 2 minutes, or until hot.
5. Pour two ¼-cup portions of pancake batter into the frying pan, and cook for about 3 minutes per side, or until lightly browned. Repeat with the remaining batter.
6. Top with honey and blueberries, if desired, and serve hot.

Moroccan Spice-Rubbed Salmon

INGREDIENTS

Rub

- 1 teaspoon garlic powder
- ½ teaspoon onion powder
- ½ teaspoon ground turmeric
- ¼ teaspoon sea salt
- ¼ teaspoon dried oregano
- ½ teaspoon garam masala or curry powder
- $1/8$ teaspoon ground ginger

Fish

- 2 (6-ounce) salmon filets
- Topping (not pictured)
- 1 small onion, sliced in rounds
- 1 tablespoon extra-virgin olive oil

INSTRUCTIONS

1. Preheat the oven to 450°F.
2. Combine all the ingredients for the rub.
3. Spread the rub on the flesh side of the salmon filets.
4. Cook the fish, without turning, for 8 minutes or until the fish flakes easily with a fork.
5. While the fish is cooking, sauté the onion in the oil. Place the sautéed onion rounds on top of the fish for the last 2 minutes of cooking.

Nutty Coconut Delight

INGREDIENTS

- ¼ cup ghee
- ½ cup raw honey
- ½ cup almonds
- 1 teaspoon cinnamon
- ¾ cup unsweetened coconut
- ½ cup walnuts, chopped

INSTRUCTIONS

1. Preheat the oven to 350°F.
2. Place the ghee, honey, almonds, and cinnamon in the bowl of a food processor fitted with a steel blade. Pulse 6 or 7 times, or until the nuts are ground.
3. Grease the bottom of an 8-inch square baking pan. Spread the nut and honey mixture over the bottom of the greased pan.
4. Sprinkle the coconut over the honey nut mixture, and then sprinkle the chopped walnuts over the coconut.
5. Place the pan in the oven and bake for 15 to 20 minutes, or until the edges bubble and begin to brown.
6. Allow the pan to cool and then refrigerate it for several hours or overnight.
7. Scoop the mixture into balls using a small ice cream scoop or serving spoon.
8. Serve immediately and refrigerate any leftovers.

Chewy Coconut Almond Cookie

INGREDIENTS

- 1 cup almond flour
- ⅓ cup unsweetened coconut
- 2 tablespoons raw honey
- 1 tablespoon coconut oil
- 1 teaspoon vanilla extract
- ¼ teaspoon almond extract
- a pinch of sea salt

INSTRUCTIONS

1. Preheat the oven to 350F
2. Place all of the ingredients into a bowl of a food processor. Pulse on and off 10 times or until the mixture begins to form a ball.
3. Line a small baking sheet with parchment paper. Divide the dough into 12 portions. Form each into a ball.
4. Place the cookies on the parchment paper and press down to flatten.
5. Bake for 8 to 10 minutes or until the edges start to brown. Do not overbake.

Creamy Asparagus Soup

INGREDIENTS

- 2 tablespoons extra virgin olive oil
- 1 medium onion, chopped
- 2 cloves garlic, chopped
- 1 large carrot, peeled and chopped
- 1 stalk celery, chopped
- 8 oz. asparagus, chopped
- 2 teaspoons freshly chopped dill
- ½ teaspoon freshly chopped tarragon
- 1 tablespoon freshly chopped parsley
- 1 teaspoon salt
- 3 cups vegetable broth
- 1 cup coconut milk

INSTRUCTIONS

1. Heat the oil in a 2-quart sauce pot over medium-high heat for 1 minute or until hot.
2. Sauté the onions for 3 minutes or until limp.
3. Add the garlic, carrots, asparagus and sauté for 5 minutes.
4. Add the remaining ingredients and stir well to combine.
5. Bring the soup to a boil over medium-high heat. Lower the heat to medium and simmer for 30 minutes.
6. Pour the soup into a blender container. Cover the container.
7. Purèe the soup until smooth.
8. Serve immediately and refrigerate leftovers.

Deviled Eggs (or Egg Salad)

INGREDIENTS

- 6 eggs, hard-boiled and peeled
- 3 tablespoons herb mayonnaise (page 271)
- 1 tablespoon mustard
- ¼ teaspoon sea salt

INSTRUCTIONS

1. Cut the peeled, cooked eggs in half lengthwise. Remove the yolks and place in a small bowl, then add the remaining ingredients. Break the yolks up with a fork and continue to mash until the mixture is smooth.

2. Spoon the filling back into the egg whites, or, if desired, pipe it back into the whites using a pastry bag fitted with a star tip.

The Root Brands Product Ingredient Index

Restore

Apple Cider Vinegar

Apple Cider Vinegar is widely used for multiple ailments and is considered a must-have in your medicine cabinet. Apple cider vinegar is a natural laxative and improves digestion, lowers blood sugar levels, lowers cholesterol, improves insulin sensitivity, aids in weight loss, reduces belly fat, lowers blood pressure, and improves heart health. It is also known to prevent and decrease the risk of getting cancer and slows down the growth of cancer cells.

Aloe Vera Gel Powder 200x

Aloe vera gel powder 200x is found in the cosmetics industry, and is also used as a supplement for GI function, but it is not limited there. Aloe vera is often deemed as "nature's miracle" because of all the things it can help. It has powerful antioxidants and anti-inflammatory properties. It aids in heart health, digestive support, liver function, and is a great nutritious boost. It is often used to clear skin, as a moisturizer and an antiseptic.

Black Cumin Seed Oil

Black seed oil is not very well known, but that doesn't mean it shouldn't be. This is a very potent oil and when its paired with antibiotics, it is capable of taking down superbugs. There are many health benefits to black seed oil, but it is often used for immune support, fighting cancer, liver health, aiding in weight loss, combating diabetes, improving acne and softening skin; it decreases asthma symptoms, reduces stomach upset, relieves headaches and toothaches, helps with parasites, wound healing, and improves rheumatoid arthritis.

Cellulose Gum

Sodium Carboxymethylcellulose, also known as sodium CMC gum, is considered to be a healthy food additive that makes foods thick and creamy, without the added fat. CMC gum is known for suppressing the appetite and is often used for weight loss diets, but otherwise offers little to no nutritional benefit.

Citric Acid

Citric Acid is one of the world's most common food additives. Often used as a preservative, people often assume it doesn't have any health benefits. Surprisingly, citric acid has anti-inflammatory and antioxidant effects, supports skin health, alkalizing, metabolizes energy, enhances nutrient absorption, and helps protect against kidney stones.

Citrus Extract

Citrus extract is an excellent source for antioxidants, vitamins, and nutrients. It is known for boosting brain health, reducing the risk of kidney stones, stabilizing blood sugar; protecting the heart, and lowering cholesterol. High in vitamin C, citrus extract supports the immune system and promotes collagen production, which helps fight wrinkles and reduce signs of aging.

D-Ribose

D-Ribose is something that the body naturally creates, but is available as a supplement. It helps support heart health, skin health, boosts energy, improves sleep, aids in mental clarity, and has anti-aging properties. Most Fibromyalgia and Chronic Fatigue Syndrome sufferers use this supplement.

Evaporated Cane Juice

Evaporated Cane Juice is a good substitute for sugar, as it sweetens foods and beverages. It's also great for baking. Unlike processed sugars, evaporated cane juice is not refined, which helps retain many of the nutrients from the cane, as well as keeping its natural tan color.

Monk Fruit Extract

Monk Fruit is one of nature's best sweeteners. It's loaded with powerful antioxidants, anti-inflammatory properties, aids in fighting cancer, fights fatigue, is a natural antihistamine, and is appropriate for low-glycemic diets due to allowing better insulin secretion.

Natural Flavors

Natural flavors is a label for substances extracted from plant or animal sources, so it is impossible to say what really goes into this ingredient. Most often, natural flavors are used to add flavor and not any nutritional value.

Zero-In

Caffeine Anhydrous

Caffeine in the nervous system clears drowsiness and gives you an energy boost. Caffeine is such an effective stimulant that many people are using a highly concentrated caffeine powder, or caffeine anhydrous, to stimulate athletic performance or weight loss. Caffeine anhydrous acts as a central nervous system stimulant by blocking the neurotransmitter adenosine's receptors, resulting in improved mood and better productivity.

L-theanine

L-theanine, an amino acid primarily found in green tea leaves, elevates levels of GABA—a natural brain relaxant—serotonin, and dopamine, and enhances alpha brain waves which may relieve anxiety and stress as well as increase focus.

N-acetyl L-tyrosine

N-acetyl L-tyrosine or NALT is a highly bioavailable form of the amino acid L-tyrosine that works in synergy with stimulants to boost dopamine, nonrepinephrine, and epinephrine levels that may increase concentration, memory, and mood.

Pine Bark Extract

Maritime pines are known to contain health-promoting plant compounds like vitamins, polyphenols, and other phytonutrients. Pine bark extract, derived from French maritime pine bark, boosts cognition and may improve alertness, memory, and mood, as well as mental flexibility and decision-making. Its other potential benefits include reducing inflammation and supporting heart health.

Turmeric Root Extract

Turmeric is argued to be one of the most powerful herbs to fight and potentially reverse disease. Health benefits range widely, but turmeric is known for being high in anti-inflammatory properties and antioxidants. Turmeric helps with boosting the immune system and mood, treating and preventing cancer, protecting the heart, healing the gut, and helping with joint pain. When it comes to brain health, turmeric or curcumin boost levels of the brain hormone BDNF, which increases the neurons, thus helping to improve memory and attention.

Velvet Bean Seed

Velvet bean seeds or Mucuna pruriens are legumes native to southern China and eastern India. Mucuna beans are very rich in minerals, essential elements, and phytonutrients. Velvet beans contain a high dose of l-dopa, a precursor to the neurotransmitter dopamine. Dopamine combined with increased serotonin and adrenaline levels may help limit Parkinson's symptoms. Velvet bean seeds also may have an anticancer effect, prevent bacterial infections, possess anti-venom properties, prevent iron deficiency, and improve mood.

Vitamin D3

Vitamin D is a nutrient your body needs for building and maintaining healthy bones. Vitamin D also regulates many other cellular functions in your body. Its anti-inflammatory, antioxidant, and neuro-protective properties support immune health, muscle function, and brain cell activity.

Clean Slate

OmniMin AC ™ Trace Minerals

Derived from the Great Salt Lake of Utah, OmniMin trace minerals include vitamins A, B, C, D, E, K, and the minerals calcium, magnesium, iron, zinc, copper, iodine, manganese, and selenium; however, ROOT's formulation has acquired over 75+ trace minerals. Trace minerals have essential functions including the following: being crucial building blocks for hundreds of enzymes, facilitating a multitude of biochemical reactions, being a requirement of normal growth and development as well as neurological functions, serving as antioxidants, and supporting the blood system.

Potassium Sorbate

Potassium sorbate is a chemical additive. It's widely used as a preservative in foods, drinks, and personal care products. It is an odorless and tasteless salt synthetically produced from sorbic acid and potassium hydroxide.

Silicon Dioxide

Silicon dioxide (SiO_2), also known as silica (derived from zeolite clinoptilolite), is a natural compound made of two of the earth's most abundant materials: silicon (Si) and oxygen (O_2). Silica may assist the body and its natural ability to promote hair, skin, and nail health, boost bone health, remove toxins and heavy metals from the body, enhance heart health, reduce digestive disorders, boost overall immune system health, accelerate the healing process, as well as potentially treat Alzheimer's disease.

Vitamin C

An essential nutrient found mainly in fruits and vegetables. The body requires vitamin C to form and maintain bones and blood vessels. It is an antioxidant that helps prevent cell damage caused by free radicals. The vitamin also helps in stimulating the immune system.

Relive Greens

Agave Americana Inulin

Agave inulin, extracted from the Agave Americana plant, is a soluble fiber and natural sweetener, supplying the body with vitamins like thiamin, niacin, folate, and B12. Agave inulin may help the body strengthen the immune system, increase production of enzymes, improve short-chain fatty acids, and reduce secretion of liver enzymes.

Alfalfa Leaf

Alfalfa leaf alkalizes and detoxifies the body due to its vitamin and mineral profile, which consists of calcium, potassium, phosphorus, iron, and vitamins A, C, E, and K. Alfalfa leaf's potential benefits on assisting the body include lowering cholesterol, improving metabolic health, reducing symptoms of diabetes, and reducing cell death and DNA damage.

Aloe Vera Gel Powder

Aloe vera is often deemed as "nature's miracle" because of all the things it can help. It has powerful antioxidants and anti-inflammatory properties. It aids in heart health, digestive support, liver function, and is a great nutritious boost. It is often used to clear skin, as a moisturizer and an antiseptic.

Apple

Apple fiber is a great source of fiber and vitamin C. They contain antioxidants, such as vitamin E and polyphenols that contribute to the fruit's numerous health benefits including assisting the body by supporting weight loss, heart function, management of diabetes, cancer prevention, asthma symptoms, and protection of the brain.

Bacilius Coagulans

Bacillus coagulans, a type of good bacteria, is a probiotic used to guard against gastrointestinal issues. Bacillus coagulans work by promoting overall gut health by removal of bad bacteria, decreasing blood pressure, improving anxiety and depression, improving sleep, shortening upper respiratory infections, lowering insulin levels, and improving cholesterol.

Barley Grass

Barley grass is rich in vitamins A and C, which act as potent antioxidants, as well as beta carotene, vitamins B1, B2, B6, B12, K, pantothenic acid, folic acid, and amino acids. This superfood may balance blood sugar levels, support heart health, promote weight loss, boost the immune system, relive ulcerative colitis, reduce signs of aging, and protect against UV radiation.

Blueberry

Blueberries possess a variety of antioxidants, fiber, and vitamins C and K. Blueberries' antioxidant contents may assist the body in neutralizing free radicals, lowering blood pressure, muscle recovery, disease protection, diabetes management, aid in weight loss, skin damage prevention, improved brain function, fight off viruses and infections, and promote heart health.

Broccoli

Broccoli consists of a number of nutrients, such as antioxidants, phytonutrients, chlorophyll, and vitamins A, B complex, K, E, as well as calcium, iron, zinc, and phosphorus. Broccoli may aid the body in preventing cancer, lowering cholesterol levels, improving vision, promoting heart health, and supporting your overall immune system.

Chlorella

Chlorella, a green-blue freshwater algae, contains a wide range of antioxidants such as omega-3s, vitamin C, and carotenoids, which may help the body's natural processes by aiding in detoxification by binding to heavy metals, enhancing the immune system, improving cholesterol, managing respiratory diseases, improving blood sugar levels as well as lowering blood pressure.

Green Banana Flour

Green banana flour, the yield of green underripe bananas, is high in essential vitamins and minerals including zinc, vitamin E, magnesium, manganese, and more. Green banana flour may assist in improving metabolism function, promoting healthy colon, aiding in weight loss, reducing insulin sensitivity, and reducing cholesterol.

Green Cabbage

Green Cabbage, a leafy vegetable belonging to the Brassica family, contains antioxidants vitamins C, K, choline, beta-carotene, and flavonoids, which work together to assist the body to improve digestion, aid in weight loss, lower cholesterol, boost immunity, reduce inflammation, heal ulcers, clear up skin, and improve cognitive function.

Jerusalem Artichoke Inulin

Jerusalem artichoke inulin is a good source of vitamins and minerals such as iron, magnesium, potassium, vitamin C, some B vitamins, fiber, and protein. Acting as a prebiotic, artichoke inulin may improve gut health, assist with blood glucose control, regulate blood pressure, reduce cholesterol, and protect against cancer.

Kale

Kale, a member of the cabbage family, is packed full of vitamins and minerals like iron, calcium, zinc, potassium, vitamins A, C, K, alpha-linolenic acid, lutein, and zeaxanthin. Its antioxidant benefits may help the body lower cholesterol, reduce risk of heart disease, fight against cancer, aid in weight loss, promote brain health, and improve eye sight.

Lactobacillus acidophilus

Lactobacillus acidophilus, one of the most common types of probiotics, balances potentially harmful bacteria that can otherwise flourish in the gut due to illness or antibiotics. It may also help prevent yeast infections. It may also assist in reducing cholesterol, preventing and reducing diarrhea, improving symptom of IBS, promoting weight loss, reducing cold and flu symptoms, preventing or reducing allergy symptoms, and/or reducing symptoms of eczema.

MCT Coconut Oil Powder

MCT coconut oil powder contains fatty acids that may fight off yeast infections and bacterial growth. Rich in vitamins E, K, and minerals such as iron, MCT coconut oil may assist the body to promote weight loss, provide energy, reduce lactate buildup, manage epilepsy, Alzheimer's disease, and autism, reduce risk factors for heart disease, and protect the liver.

Parsley

Parsley, a fresh herb, is very bountiful in vitamins A, K, potassium, as well as vitamin C, folate, and phosphorus. Parsley's potential benefits may support optimal functioning of the body by improving blood sugar, promoting heart health, aiding in kidney health, fighting against bacteria, boosting the immune system, and enhancing liver health.

Pomegranate Seed Powder

Pomegranate Seed Powder is rich in fiber, antioxidants, and fatty acids as well as vitamin E and magnesium. Pomegranate seeds may help the body fight against prostate and breast cancers, lower blood pressure, fight arthritis and joint pain, lower risk of heart disease, ward off bacterial and fungal infections, improve memory, and improve exercise performance.

Psyllium Husk Powder

Psyllium husk powder, a type of dietary fiber from the Plantago ovata plant, may support the body's ability to decrease blood glucose, encourage weight loss, lower blood pressure, help with healthy bowel movements, lower cholesterol, and overall act as a natural laxative.

Spinach

Spinach, a dark leafy vegetable rich in vitamins A, C, and E, possesses antioxidant and anti-cancer properties. It's other potential benefits include promoting bone mass, fighting against inflammation, preventing cancer, improving vision, preventing or managing degenerative diseases, aiding in weight loss, promoting healthy digestion, and aiding in detoxification of the colon.

Spirulina

Spirulina, a blue-green algae, is packed full of antioxidants, minerals, chlorophyll, and phycocyanins that may assist the body by aiding in weight loss, improving gut health, managing diabetes, lowering cholesterol, managing blood pressure, preventing heart disease, boosting metabolism, reducing fatigue, and promoting cell regeneration.

Wheat Grass

Wheat Grass, derived from the Triticum aestivum plant, contains a variety of nutrients such as vitamins, minerals, amino acids, chlorophyll, and proteins. Wheat grass's nutritional profile may support the body and its natural ability to eliminate toxins, aid digestion, boost metabolism, strengthen immune system, improve cognitive function, ease joint pain, and improve energy.

Natural Barrier Support

Vitamin C

An essential nutrient found mainly in fruits and vegetables. The body requires vitamin C to form and maintain bones and blood vessels. It is an antioxidant that helps prevent cell damage caused by free radicals. The vitamin also helps in stimulating the immune system.

Mitochondria Shield Defense

B-Nicotinamide Adenine Dinucleotide (NAD+)

NAD+ (nicotinamide adenine dinucleotide) is a coenzyme found in all living cells that is essential in key physiological processes in our bodies. As we get older, however, NAD+ production slows down, leading to mental and physical fatigue. NAD+ may reverse the aging processes, improve cognitive function, assist in weight management, boost energy, aid in muscle development and recovery, support pain management, improve overall mood, and improve cardiovascular health.

Magnesium

From regulating blood sugar levels to boosting athletic performance, magnesium is crucial for your brain and body. Magnesium is found all throughout your body; in fact, every cell in your body contains this mineral and needs it to function. It's involved in more than 600 reactions in your body, including energy creation, protein formation, gene maintenance, muscle movements, and nervous system regulation.

OmniMin AC ™ Trace Minerals

Derived from the Great Salt Lake of Utah, OmniMin trace minerals includes vitamins A, B, C, D, E, K, and the minerals calcium, magnesium, iron, zinc, copper, iodine, manganese, and selenium; however, ROOT's formulation has acquired over 75+ trace minerals. Trace minerals have essential functions including the following: being crucial building blocks for hundreds of enzymes, facilitating a multitude of biochemical reactions, being a requirement of normal growth and development as well as neurological functions, serving as antioxidants, and supporting the blood system.

Quercetin

Quercetin is a plant pigment (flavonoid) with powerful antioxidant and anti-inflammatory effects. Quercetin is most commonly used for conditions of the heart and blood vessels and to prevent cancer. It is also used for arthritis, bladder infections, and diabetes. People take quercetin for serval reasons, including to boost immunity, fight inflammation, reverse the aging processes, combat allergy, aid exercise performance, and maintain overall general health.

Vitamin D3

Vitamin D is a nutrient your body needs for building and maintaining healthy bones. Vitamin D also regulates many other cellular functions in your body. Its anti-inflammatory, antioxidant, and neuroprotective properties support immune health, muscle function, and brain cell activity.

Zinc Sulfate

Zinc is important for growth and for the development and health of the body's tissues. Zinc sulfate boosts your body's zinc levels and prevents and treats deficiency. You need zinc for a robust immune system, because it makes up a component of enzymes that help trigger an immune response as well as hormones needed for immune cell function.

Hydrolyzed Bovine Collagen

Collagen, found in your body and numerous animals, is an abundant source of protein. It serves as one of the major building blocks in skin, bones, tendons, ligaments, muscles, and blood vessels. Bovine collagen is a form of this protein that's mainly derived from cows. Bovine collagen has been found to increase types I and III collagen. The collagen in your skin is primarily made up of types I and III collagen, meaning that bovine collagen may be especially useful for reducing wrinkles, promoting elasticity, and increasing skin moisture.

Whole Colostrum Powder

Colostrum is a breast fluid produced by humans, cows, and other mammals before breast milk is released. It's very nutritious and contains high levels of antibodies, which are proteins that fight infections and bacteria. Even though all mammals produce colostrum, supplements are usually made from the colostrum of cows. This supplement is known as bovine colostrum.

Bovine colostrum contains macronutrients, vitamins, and minerals. It's especially high in protein compounds that regulate immune responses and promote growth, including lactoferrin, growth factors, and antibodies. Colostrum may boost immunity, strengthen gut health, and promote overall digestive health.

Vitamin C

An essential nutrient found mainly in fruits and vegetables. The body requires vitamin C to form and maintain bones and blood vessels. It is an antioxidant that helps prevent cell damage caused by free radicals. The vitamin also helps in stimulating the immune system.

Vitamin D

Vitamin D is a nutrient your body needs for building and maintaining healthy bones. Vitamin D also regulates many other cellular functions in your body. Its anti-inflammatory, antioxidant, and neuroprotective properties support immune health, muscle function, and brain cell activity.

Vitamin K2

Vitamin K is important in the blood coagulation process via the modification of protein molecules. Several studies have reported more health benefits with vitamin K2 than with vitamin K1. It contributes to skin health and bone metabolism, promotes proper brain function, and prevents heart-related diseases. Furthermore, vitamin K2 is important in the body's use of calcium to help build bones and to inhibit blood vessel calcification.

CPSIA information can be obtained
at www.ICGtesting.com
Printed in the USA
LVHW070553250123
737623LV00001B/6